W9-CFE-089

TABLE
OF CONTENTS

INTRODUCTION

We all know a thinner body is not only a more attractive body, but it is also a healthier body. We feel less self conscious, we have more energy, and we enjoy participating more in life. A thinner body is more agile and athletic. A thinner body has more sex appeal!

How often have you promised yourself that by next summer, "I will wear that bikini bathing suit." How often have you wished you had a thinner more attractive body? Let's face the facts—"looking good is feeling good." Our self image has a tremendous effect on our moods. Our moods (anxieties, fears, depressions), affect our behavior. One of our most obvious behaviors is eating. It becomes a vicious cycle. A poor self image can lead to excessive worry, which can lead to overeating!!

How many times have you asked yourself, "Why can't I find a diet that really works, so I can look thinner?" You may say, "I lose weight, but I can never keep it off!" Weight reduction is not always weight loss. If the weight is gained back only a few weeks after the strenuous dieting, what have you really achieved?

Virginia Aronson has now presented an intelligent alternative to Diet Plans. In *The Joy of Being Thin,* she reveals the secret to successful weight *loss.* The answer lies in 1) understanding, 2) insight, and 3) modification of your eating habits. She presents an analytic and thought-provoking look at why people eat. By helping us to understand our reactions and emotions to food, we can begin to change our "fat habits" to "health habits".

Eating to most people is a pleasurable psychological experience. We know that we don't always eat because we feel hunger. Sometimes we eat from emotions like boredom, tension, or depression. The "Twelve New Health

Habits", are specifically designed to give you control over your emotions, rather than letting your emotions control you.

The 30 Day Menu Plan is exciting and varied, to assist you in deriving the psychological benefits from eating, without feeling deprived. In addition, the reader is provided with a Calorie Listing for over 1,000 foods—a handy reference guide.

Get yourself "psyched up" for some interesting reading and sensible weight loss, as you prepare yourself for the "Thinner You"!!

—Dr. Neil H. Edison

Dr. Neil H. Edison is a Diplomate of the American Boards of Psychiatry and Neurology, practicing in Miami, Florida. He studied at Cornell Medical Center of New York and Beth Israel Hospital of New York. Currently, Dr. Edison is Chairman of the Dept. of Psychiatry at North Miami General Hospital.

Virginia Aronson, the author of "The Joy Of Being Thin", is an extremely talented registered dietitian with a Master's degree in nutrition. She is the author of several books, including "Guide Book For Nutrition Counselors", a newly released textbook on nutrition. Currently, Ms. Aronson is conducting dietary research at Harvard University.

FAT HABITS—AND HOW TO CHANGE THEM

ORAL ABUSE DEFINED

Are you an oral abuser? There are three major oral abuses people tend to inflict upon themselves:

a. cigarette smoking
b. excessive drinking of alcoholic beverages
c. overeating

These are planned abuses, and can lead to a variety of well-known health problems. Oral abusers tend to have higher than normal incidences of:

a. lung cancer
b. emphysema
c. oral cancers
d. respiratory disorders
e. cirrhosis
f. pancreatitis
g. nutritional deficiencies
h. heart disease
i. diabetes
j. gall bladder dysfunctions
k. fertility and pregnancy problems
l. premature aging and early death

An impressively fearful and probably familiar list, yet many individuals ignore the medical facts and continue along their paths of self-destruction. Why? They feel *compelled* to.

A compulsion is an uncontrollable psychological drive to do something, oftentimes abusive. When eating becomes a compulsion, like smoking and drinking, the oral abuser feels *compelled* to overindulge. Unlike smoking and drinking, however, the oral abuser cannot stop "cold turkey" (although starvation is actually easier for some indivudals, for whom a biteful inevitably results in a binge).

Overeating on occassion is not seriously abusive. In comparison, neither the annual New Year's Eve celebration nor a week of teenage experimentation with cigarettes can be considered to be seriously self-destructive. But many people are totally unaware of what food means to them individually and of how they personally use food. It is this lack of insight which can prove to be both abusive and unhealthy.

You need to start to gain insight, so that you can increase your awareness of your own personal food habits. Determining why you do what you do is a complex process, but even a small degree of insight can result in valuable self-improvement.

FOOD HABIT INSIGHT: QUIZ YOURSELF

From infancy on, each individual develops specific habits and shapes personal views. Eating patterns are also influenced by the way each individual leads his or her life. And everyone has personal feelings about the emotional aspects of eating, the meaning of food, and the psychological effects of diet.

What are *your* feelings about food and you? Why do you eat as you do? Try to use some true insight in answering the following SELF QUIZ questions; take several minutes for honest self-reflection prior to checking (✓) the appropriate answers for each.

FOOD HABITS SELF-QUIZ

Never	Seldom	Often		
____	____	____	1.	Do you reward yourself with food?
____	____	____	2.	Do you eat everything on your plate?

___	___	___	3.	Do you associate certain people, places, events from the past with specific foods?
___	___	___	4.	Does the sight of food make you feel hungry?
___	___	___	5.	Does the smell of food make you feel hungry?
___	___	___	6.	Does the thought of food make you feel hungry?
___	___	___	7.	Do you eat according to the clock (e.g. noon means lunchtime)?
___	___	___	8.	Do you eat while engaged in other activities (e.g. reading, watching T.V., working, driving, talking on the phone, etc.)?
___	___	___	9.	Do you eat when you are feeling emotional (e.g. bored, frustrated, nervous, lonely, depressed, happy, tense, etc.)?
___	___	___	10.	So you delay or avoid unpleasant activities by eating instead.?
___	___	___	11.	Do you eat due to the influence of others?
___	___	___	12.	Do you find yourself seeking (unsuccessfully) foods that you think will satisfy you?

Read on to further your own understanding of yourself, your personal food habits, your "fat habits". Perhaps you can make some constructive changes.

FAT HABITS FROM THE PAST

Every individual develops different eating behaviors, partially due to different upbringings. You now have certain food habits which have been instilled in you since infancy, childhood, your teen years or early adulthood. Your parents have had much to do with the development of your food habits, as have other relatives and friends. Whether your food habits are fat habits can in part be traced to your past.

Do you reward yourself with food? In other words, do you find yourself reaching for cookies and milk when you:

    a. have had a difficult day at work?
    b. have had a troublesome day with the children?
    c. are not feeling well, physically?
    d. have been dieting for awhile with success?
    e. have been dieting for awhile without success?
    f. receive a promotion?
    g. pass an exam?
    h. feel that you deserve a break?

Can you recall whether your parents rewarded you with food? Do you remember them giving you cookies and milk when you:

    a. brought home good grades?
    b. went to bed when asked?
    c. stopped fighting or crying?
    d. were well-behaved?

Do you reward others with food? Do you find yourself offering someone cookies and milk when they:

    a. do what you tell them to do?
    b. complain of having had a difficult day?
    c. cry, or are physically or emotionally hurt?
    d. are well-behaved?

In all of the situations mentioned above, food is not used as a *physical* means to rid hunger, but as a *psychological* "lift". If you use food to reward yourself or others, you tend to develop special meanings for food, and associate feeling emotionally lifted with eating food. With life today as we know it, it is no wonder that over one-third of the American population is overweight: inflation, world problems, divorce, child-rearing, rioting, illness, wars, crime...many look to food to supply that needed emotional lift. Do you?

Do you eat everything on your plate? This habit is appropriately known as the "clean plate" syndrome. If you were forced to habitually clean your plate as a child, perhaps even punished when you refused, you may find yourself compulsed to still do so. This means that you:

a. feel guilty if you cannot finish a meal.
b. rarely leave even a single bite of food on your plate.
c. force others to finish their food.
d. give yourself/others dessert ONLY when everything has been eaten.
e. eat leftovers from others' plates, rather than have food "go to waste".

Habits instilled in the early years are especially difficult to change. Yet sometimes they can be replaced by healthier, more sensible habits. If you really think about it, isn't it more wasteful and less sensible for you to overeat to the point of discomfort and eventual overweight, than it is for you to dispose of unneeded food? So what if you scrape a few mouthfuls of casserole into the garbage? Isn't that less wastefull than adding more to your full waist?

Do you associate certain people, places, events from the past with specific foods? In other words, does food mean more to you than simply a cure for physical hunger? For example, because of your own particular past history:

a. eating chicken soup reminds you of being comforted by your loving grandmother.
b. a trip to the seacoast always includes a pint of fried clams.

9

c. dinner is never over until dessert has been
      devoured.
   Again, the habits you developed in your earlier years
may now be undertaken without forethought, and difficult for you to break. Identification of the fat habits,
your faulty eating behaviors, is the first step toward making the necessary changes. Your past is an important
component in the present YOU, but must you allow your
past to determine your present decisions? Do you want
your past mistakes to mis-shape your present and future
self?

CHANGE YOUR FAT HABITS FROM THE PAST

   Your past has a definite, strong influence over your
current decisions and state of being. Since today is the
first day in the rest of your being, why not start now—and
make your *own* decisions? Rather than try to totally
eliminate your past influences, learn to recognize them
for what they are, and control them. You can control your
present, and not let your past control you!
   Start today by incorporating the following suggestions
into your daily eating patterns. Once you have adopted
THE JOY OF BEING THIN DIET PLAN, and have adhered
to THE COMPLETE 30-DAY JOY OF BEING THIN MENU
PLAN, these habit changes will have become routine! It
is quite difficult to break old habits, but it becomes
easier if you actually *replace* these fat habits—with different, healthier habits.
   HEALTH HABIT NO. 1: Choose desirable alter-
   natives to food for use as a reward (e.g. after a difficult day, reward yourself with a relaxing bath or
   reward your spouse for a promotion with tickets to
   a popular show).
   HEALTH HABIT NO. 2: Leave one bite of food on
   your plate at each meal or snack, and stop forcing
   others to eat against their will. (Buy a leftovers

10

cookbook and/or get used to the idea that overeating is more wasteful/waist-full than disposing of extra food).

HEALTH HABIT NO. 3: Whenever you are eating, ask yourself this question—am I eating by choice, or due to someone, someplace, some event from my past?

(Remember, identification is the first step toward change!)

These are the first of 12 HEALTH HABITS which you will learn to utilize to your advantage. Eventually, your habits will support your good health and thin self. You are on your way to enjoying the thin life!

FAT HABITS DUE TO ENVIRONMENT

Your eating habits are highly susceptible to outside influences. There are multiple "cues" existing in the world around you which influence your eating behaviors. Many people learn to respond only to these outside, *external* eating cues, rather than to their own physical *internal* feelings of hunger. It is important to be able to distinguish between the two, so that you can learn to eat in response to *internal* hunger rather than because of *external* influences.

Does the sight of food make you feel hungry? In other words, do you find yourself:

a. running to the kitchen for a snack after seeing a television commercial for chocolate chip cookies?
b. drooling at the mere sight of an ice cream shop?
c. dry and parched after passing a billboard for frosty cold beer?
d. making a special trip to the local baker after catching a glimpse of plump blueberry muffins in a cookbook or magazine?

When you eat in response to the sight of food, rather than because you are physically hungry, you are responding falsely. You are allowing your environment to manipulate your eating behaviors and thereby make food choices for you. Shouldn't YOU be the one to decide when and what YOU eat?

Does the smell of food make you hungry? A large percentage of how a food tastes comes from its odor. Yet, the mere aroma of edible items is not a true indication of physical need. Do you find that:

a. whenever you are roasting meat, your nose tempts you into nibbling?
b. if you walk past a bakery, the aroma of freshly baked bread always draws you inside?
c. you can never pass up a bucket of popcorn at the movie theater, once the odor has entered your nostrils?

Again, you are allowing the environment around you to determine whether you are to eat, or not eat—and what you will eat. It should be your mind and your body together which make the decision, rather than your world manipulating its intended reaction from you.

Does the thought of food make you feel hungry? In other words, do you find yourself:

a. fantasizing over hot fundge sundaes and hot, buttered rolls everytime you go on a diet?
b. dreaming about eating rich, heavy, gourmet feasts?
c. unable to control your thoughts about food so that eventually they monopolize your mind and you can only halt the tortuous process by eating?

Quite often an external trigger can lock your mind in the refrigerator! Do not let your environment trap you in cold storage! You can control your thoughts, instead of allowing them to have control over you. And you can control your eating habits, instead of letting them have control over you.

Do you eat according to the clock? Time should not be the decision maker as to whether you eat or not. For you, do the following statements ring true?

a. Noon is a four letter word for lunch.
b. Six o'clock signals cocktails and hors d'oeuvres.
c. Coffee break means coffee. And donuts.
d. Bedtime could be accurately renamed "snacktime".

When you eat in response to time rather than eating when you are physically hungry, you are responding to the external and ignoring the internal. Many people become so structured in their eating schedules, that they lose touch with their own internal hunger signs. Can you recognize *your* internal hunger cues?

Do you eat while engaged in other activities? In other words, do you:
a. devour your eggs and bacon while reading the morning newspaper?
b. munch, munch, munch whenever you watch television?
c. chew on candies to help you complete the boring household chores?
d. stretch your phone cord to the refrigerator so that you can eat and talk at the same time?
e. keep candy in the glove compartment of your car?
f. think that a weekend of television sports without peanuts and beer would be an outright sin?

Often when the mind is occupied with one activity, a simultaneous activity is not fully assimilated. This is why you may find that you have consumed all of your popcorn during a movie without even realizing that you have done so; it sometimes seems as if someone else must have taken your food! When you fail to concentrate on eating as a sole activity, you may not derive the psychological benefits of eating—and you end up unconsciously and consciously, eating *more* than you think, need, or want to eat.

Food can bring us great psychological pleasure. But if you eat while your mind is concentrating elsewhere, the psychological satisfaction is lost, causing your psyche to urge you to eat more.

CHANGE YOUR ENVIRONMENTALLY INDUCED FAT HABITS

The world around you has considerable influence over the decisions you make and the actions you undertake. It is up to you to recognize environmental eating cues, and to learn to deal with them. You can control your environment and avoid allowing it to manipulate you!

Begin now by incorporating the following suggestions into your daily eating patterns. Once you have adopted THE JOY OF BEING THIN DIET PLAN, and have adhered to THE COMPLETE 30-DAY JOY OF BEING THIN MENU PLAN, these habit changes will have become routine! Again, it is hard to break old habits, but it becomes less difficult if you actually *replace* these fat habits—with new, healthier habits.

HEALTH HABIT NO. 4: Whenever you *see* something which tempts you to eat, STOP—wait 10 minutes, during which time you should try to determine whether you are physically hungry; eat the tempting food ONLY if you feel that you are physically hungry, and if NO other substitute will do. Eat only *half* of the amount which you are tempted to eat.

HEALTH HABIT NO. 5: Whenever you *smell* something which tempts you to eat, STOP—wait for 10 minutes, during which time you should try to determine whether you are physically hungry; eat the tempting food ONLY if you feel that you are physically hungry, and if NO other substitute will do. Eat only *half* of the amount which you are tempted to eat.

HEALTH HABIT NO. 6: Whenever you *think* of some food which tempts you to eat, STOP—wait for 10 minutes, during which time you should try to determine whether you are physically hungry; eat the tempting food ONLY if you feel that you are physically hungry, and if NO other substitute will do. Eat only *half* of the amount which you are tempted to eat.

HEALTH HABIT NO. 7: Whenever you are about to eat because it is time to eat, STOP—wait for 10 minutes, during which time you should try to determine whether you are physically hungry; eat ONLY if you feel that you are physically hungry.

HEALTH HABIT NO. 8: Make eating a sole activity. This means that when you are eating, do ONLY that; no more eating while reading, watching television, working, talking on the phone, etc. In order to ease this change in habits, remove food from the areas where you usually engage in other activities; keep food *inside* the kitchen, and your activities *outside* the kitchen. It may also be helpful to choose a habitual eating place (e.g. A.M.—dining room table, LUNCH—cafeteria, P.M.—dining room table) and do *all* of your eating there.

These 5 HEALTH HABITS can assist you in taking control of your environment, rather than allowing it to control you. You are on your way to full control over your eating behaviors, your health and weight, yourself!

FAT HABITS AND YOUR EMOTIONS

Every individual has a variety of personal feelings about food. Food represents different things to different people, and influences each person in a separate way. You eat food for a multitude of reasons, and it is your own responsibility to determine these reasons to thereby understand your own particular food habits. Remember, identification can lead to constructive change!

Do you eat when you are feeling emotional? Whether your emotions are pleasant, unpleasant, or confused, do you drown your feelings in a sea of food? Do you find that:

a. when you are bored, a sandwich provides
   something to do?
b. if family frustrations get you down, a few cookies
   will help to lift your spirits?
c. whenever traffic leads to tension, a candy bar or a
   few mints can calm you down?
d. you cry into your soup, and rejoice into your ice
   cream sundae?

Food does serve many important emotional functions,
including:

a. relieving boredom.
b. easing frustration.
c. soothing tense nerves.
d. providing friendship.
e. cheering woes.
f. helping to enhance celebration.

Unfortuantely for food-lovers, food can only serve
these functions TEMPORARILY. Food does not provide a
cure, but merely a means for delay in dealing wth problems and emotions. You probably will not solve your
marital problems with an anchovy pizza, nor can you
clear up your financial difficulties with a dozen donuts. In
fact, you may add to your personal problems by choosing
to eat rather than to deal with yourself.

Do you delay or avoid unpleasant activities by eating
instead? In other words, do you:

a. opt for a trip to the local ice cream parlor instead of
   tackling the overgrown lawn?
b. find yourself taking several coffee (and donut)
   breaks during particularly dull or difficult work
   days?
c. put off making the necessary but unpleasant phone
   call for an hour or so and make a giant sandwich instead?
d. prefer (and usually choose) sharing hamburgers
   and shakes with your friends over doing homework

alone in the library?

Food can serve as an excellent substitute for less pleasurable tasks, and eating is always an enjoyable—if only temporary—diversion. Food is too easily and too often used in order to avoid confrontation, to escape from duties, and to avoid dealing with oneself. Do you use food in this way?

Do you eat due to the influence of others? Your friends, family, relatives, even enemies have a great deal to do with what, when, and why you eat. Do you find that:

a. a visit from your mother-in-law is tolerable only when accompanied by milk chocolate?

b. your spouse drives you to pasta, your children drive you to pastry, and your neighbors drive you to pasta, pastry, and pineapple pie?

c. you always overindulge when your friend "Let's-eat-a-lot-Charlie" is around.

d. the girls always force you to have Danish and coffee; the boys always force you to have ham sandwiches and beer?

e. a broken relationship invariably leads to a broken diet?

f. a visit to the parents inevitably leads to an earful and a bellyful?

People certainly can trigger one's emotions, and emotions can influence eating behaviors. By determining *who* results in *which* eating response, you may learn how to control *yourself*—even if others seem unable to control *themselves* around you! And there is nothing unhealthy in avoiding "problem" people during especially emotional periods, and dieting is often a time of heightened emotions.

Do you find yourself seeking (unsuccessfully) foods that you think will satisfy you? Can you think of frustrating times when you:

a. nibbled on 13 pickles, 2 tossed salads, 1 pint of cot-

tage cheese, 10 melba toasts, assorted fruits, and
several "light" beers, before you realized that you
really wanted to go out for dinner instead?
b. gobbled down 4 different varieties of chocolate
bars, yet still did not find the kind you *really*
wanted?
c. really needed attention, but fixed yourself an onion
omelette instead?
d. find yourself with your head in the refrigerator, your
face in the kitchen cabinets, your hand in the
cookie jar—but you do not have any idea what you
are searching for?

Before you can successfully satisfy your needs, you
must determine why you want to eat and what your exact
needs are. Insight and self-awareness can mean the dif
ference between a dissatisfying food binge and a prob
lem solved!

THE JOY OF BEING THIN DIET PLAN

WHY THIS DIET PLAN?

Excess body weight is not only unattractive, but it is a
health hazard as well. Most people are well aware of the
physical complications and emotional difficulties which
accompany overweight, yet over one third of the
American population carries extra poundage—and
repeatedly fails in attempts to rid themselves of it. This is
due to the popular outlook that diet is a temporary cure
for overweight, rather than a lifelong means for maintain
ing good health and desired body shape.

Many dieters fail to achieve their dieting goals
because they are unrealistic in their expectations. Crash
diets are quite popular, despite being commonly unsuc
cessful in the long run. Based on impractical and tem
porary goals, crash diets appeal to most dieters because
they boast of fantastic results with relatively little effort

n extraordinary short periods of time. The numerous variety of crash diets available on the market today offers dieters a lifetime of different diet plans to try. How many of the following crash diets have YOU experimented with?

a. High protein diet
b. Liquid protein diet
c. Low protein diet
d. High carbohydrate diet
e. Low carbohydrate diet
f. No carbohydrate diet
g. Dr. Stillman's diet
h. Dr. Atkin's diet
i. Air Force diet
j. Ski Team diet
k. Drinking Man's diet
l. Water diet
m. Fruit and rice diet
n. Macrobiotic diet
o. Cottage cheese and bananas diet
p. Eggs and tomato diet
q. Hot dogs and grapefruit diet
r. Ice cream lovers' diet
s. Diet for lovers
t. Liquid diet
u. Fasting diet
v. Starvation diet
w. The Last Diet

The diets may appear to be different, yet the theme is the same: restricted caloric intake, without regard to nutrient content, for quick but temporary losses of body weight. Most of the initial weight loss is not of body fat, but of body *fluids;* because body fluids weigh as much as body fat, the scales show an inspiring decline in weight...which returns as soon as old eating habits (FAT HABITS) are resumed. And due to the repetitious and dissatisfying contents of the typical crash diet, most dieters are unable to adhere to the diet plan long enough to reach desired weight loss goals.

Crash diets also share another deceitful trait: they do nothing to assist the dieter in making food habit changes. By offering merely a temporary means for rapid weight loss, these diets fail to teach the dieter how to eat once the diet is completed. Crash dieters do not increase their awareness concerning their own individual food habits. Remember, identification is the first step toward change—and it is only *permanent* habit changes which are able to support *permanent* weight losses.

THE JOY OF BEING THIN DIET PLAN is low enough in calories to allow for quick, yet safe weight loss. The DIET PLAN is restricted in calorie content, yet provides essential nutrients if followed properly. If you follow crash diets, or eliminate foods from THE JOY OF BEING THIN DIET in hopes of speeding up your weight loss rate, you will probably not obtain all of the nutritive ingredients necessary for proper body function. This can lead to:

a. irritability, depression, nervousness
b. headache
c. weakness, dizziness
d. fatique
e. other symptoms of caloric-nutrient deficiencies

CALORIES EXPLAINED

Calories are a unit of measure, an amount of heat, and are used to express the energy provided by food. If a food is high in calories, it provides you with a lot of energy. If a food is low in calories, then it provides little energy. Your body needs a certain amount of energy each day so that you can function at your best. If you take in too much energy (too many calories), the extra will be stored as body fat. If you do not take in enough food energy to meet your needs (too few calories), then you will lose body fat.

This balance is a simple formula:

 a. EXCESS CALORIES = TOO MUCH ENERGY = STORED BODY FAT = WEIGHT GAIN
 b. INADEQUATE CALORIES = USE OF BODY FAT FOR ENERGY = WEIGHT LOSS

It is this latter balance which THE JOY OF BEING THIN DIET PLAN can achieve for you...all *you* have to do is to follow the DIET and MENU PLAN, carefully and accurately. Your caloric intake will be low, yet your nutritional status will not suffer. In fact, it may improve!

The key number is 3500—there are 3500 calories in one pound of body fat. In order to GAIN one pound of body fat, you must take in 3500 calories MORE than your body needs. And in order to LOSE one pound of body fat, you must take in 3500 calories LESS than your body requires.

You need not create a 3500 calorie deficit in a single day. Instead, you can spread out your total caloric decrease and subsequent weight loss over several days...a week...a month...a year. If you lower your caloric intake by 500 calories per day, you should lose one pound in a week (500 x 7 = 3500 or one pound). This can result in a 4-5 pound weight loss in a single month (one pound/week x 4-5 = 4-5 pounds). And after a year, the total weight loss will be over 50 pounds (one pound/week x 52 weeks = 52 pounds)!

If you want to lose weight more rapidly than illustrated above, you would need to increase your caloric deficit beyond 500 calories; with a 1000 calorie daily deficit, 2 pounds can be lost per week, and with a 1500 calorie daily deficit, 3 pounds can be lost each week.

Weigh yourself once a week ONLY, in the morning, without clothing. Each week record your weight in the PERSONAL WEIGHT CHART ON PAGE 48. By graphing your weight, you are also able to visualize your weekly rate of weight loss.

There is no need to try to hasten your weight loss rate.

21

THE JOY OF BEING THIN DIET PLAN allows for rapid loss of excess weight, safely and effectively, while simultaneously assisting you in adopting new eating behaviors—HEALTHY HABITS.

Why risk diet failure and all the physical and psychological distrubances which accompany this plight, when adherence to this well-balanced DIET PLAN and gradual adoption of a few simple new food habits can result in a thinner, healthier, happier you? And you can begin right now, with THE JOY OF BEING THIN DIET PLAN. What have YOU got to lose?

YOUR DIET DIARY

Another helpful habit is to continuously record all food eaten in a DIET DIARY. It is important to record everything *immediately* following consumption for two reasons:

a. If you wait until the days' end, you may forget to record certain foods you have eaten, especiall snacks and nibbles.

b. The knowledge that you must write down each item eaten may help you to resist impulsive eating.

Begin keeping a DIET DIARY; ample space is provided in the APPENDIX (see pages 127, 128). Try to be quit descriptive in your entries: give details concerning each food and beverage consumed, measure and record exact amounts, and describe any feelings or emotions you may experience relative to your food habits and the DIET PLAN itself. Specific details can provide you with vivid recollections of:

a. *what* exactly you are consuming.

b. *how much* you consume.

c. how you *feel* about your consumption habits.

Try to be as honest as possible with yourself when you record in your DIET DIARY. Failure to include foods eaten or to record true feelings will only serve to prevent you from developing insight and food habit awareness.

If utilized properly, your DIET DIARY can serve as an effective means for:

   a. revealing actual quantities of your food intake.
   b. providing insight into your own personal eating habits.
   c. changing diet and eating behaviors—from FAT HABITS to HEALTH HABITS—and for observing these changes.

Since you are going to start on THE JOY OF BEING THIN DIET PLAN today (or tomorrow at the latest), you should begin keeping track of your food intake immediately. See how closely you can adhere to THE COMPLETE 30-DAY JOY OF BEING THIN MENU PLAN. The less deviations or substitutions you make in the MENU PLAN, the better your results will be. Too many alterations in the DIET or MENU PLANS can lead to outright failure in your weight loss goals. Instead, you might:

   a. feel psychological deprivation from the exclusion of certain necessary foods.
   b. mistakenly include high-calorie foods.
   c. alter the balance of the DIET PLAN.
   d. DISCONTINUE THE JOY OF BEING THIN DIET PLAN at an early date.
   e. fail to improve both your food habits and your figure.

THE JOY OF BEING THIN DIET PLAN

THE JOY OF BEING THIN DIET PLAN IS A complete guide to well-balanced, low-calorie eating. It is rich in nutrient content, and includes a wide variety of delicious, health-promoting foods. Simply by following the COMPLETE 30-DAY JOY OF BEING THIN MENU PLAN, you can lose weight while you adopt new food habits. By the month's end, your FAT HABITS should be modified, while HEALTH HABITS will have become routine.

THE JOY OF BEING THIN DIET PLAN includes th
following:
BREAKFAST—
   Approximately 250 calories
LUNCH—
   Approximately 350 caloires
DINNER—
   Approximately 400 calories
SNACK (optional)—
   Approximately 200 calories
TOTALS—
   Approximately 1000 calories per day
   Approximately 1200 calories per day, including SNAC
NOTE: Meal totals may vary from day to day, but TOTAL
are accurate for all days.

So, simply follow THE COMPLETE 30-DAY JOY OF BE
ING THIN MENU PLAN. It has been designed to fit TH
JOY OF BEING THIN DIET PLAN, so be sure to adhere t
THE MENU PLAN carefully and accurately. Deviation
and substitutions could alter the TOTALS and subse
quently result in undesirable effects on your diet goals

Once the initial 30 days are over, you should b
familiar with both low-calorie eating and the HEALTH
HABITS which accompany your new diet plan. Use the
LISTING COUNTER and PLANNING COUNTER beginning
on page 53 to assist you in devising your own low-calorie
health-promoting menus. If you dine out, follow the sug
gestions outlined in DINING OUT DO'S AND DON'T'S o
page 44 in order to make appropriate food selections.

THE JOY OF BEING THIN can help you to gain insigh
into your own personal food habits and to develop ar
understanding of the changes necessary for an improvec
diet. With the adequate knowledge and self
responsibility, your FAT HABITS will become HEALTH
HABITS, and you will be on your way to a thinner
healther, happier you.

THE COMPLETE 30-DAY JOY OF BEING THIN
MENU PLAN

Remember to follow the MENU PLAN as closely as possible and to record your intake in your DIET DIARY (see APPENDIX). Enjoy!

DAY ONE

Breakfast: 1/2 cup pineapple juice
1/4 cup grape nuts with
1/3 cup skim milk and
1/2 banana, sliced

Lunch: 1 whole wheat bagel broiled with
1-1/2 oz. part skim mozzarella cheese and
1/4 cup sliced mushrooms
1 cup fresh strawberries

Dinner: 4 oz. broiled cod
1 sm. boiled potato with
1 tsp. margarine
sliced tomatoes broiled with
2tbsp. grated parmesan cheese
tossed salad with low-cal dressing

Snack: 1 sm. slice carrot cake

DAY TWO

Breakfast: 1/2 cup grapefruit juice
1 cup puffed wheat cereal with
1/2 cup skim milk sprinkled with
1 tbsp. each: wheat germ, chopped
walnuts, unprocessed bran

Lunch: Salade Nicoise—
1 cup lettuce, bite-size
1 sm. artichoke heart, quartered
1/2 cup green beans
1 cup assorted vegies
1 tbsp. low-calorie Italian dressing
3 whole wheat bread sticks
1 dried fig

Dinner: 3-1/2 oz. dry white wine
4 oz. broiled chicken
1/2 cup brown rice with
1 tbsp. slivered almonds
1/2 cup broccoli
tossed salad with low-cal dressing

Snack: 1 cup low fat yogurt with
3/4 cup fresh blueberries

DAY THREE

Breakfast: 1/2 cup tangerine sections
1 egg omelet made with
1/4 cup sliced tomato, pepper, onion and
1/2 oz. part-skim cheese
1 whole wheat English muffin

Lunch: Tuna pocket (bake in foil)—
1 mini whole wheat pita pocket stuffed w/
1/2 cup tuna fish
2 tsp. low-cal mayonnaise
3 tbsp. chopped celery, onion, pepper
1 oz. pat-skim mozzarella cheese
1 sm. fresh peach

Dinner: Spinach Pasta Bake (bake until bubbly)—
3/4 cup spinach pasta, cooked al dente
1/2 cup cottage cheese, uncreamed
1/4 cup low-fat yogurt
1 oz. part-skim mozzarella cheese, shredded
assorted seasonings to taste
1 sm. whole wheat roll
tossed salad with low-cal dressing

Snack: 1/4 cup raisins mixed with
1/8 cup unsalted peanuts

DAY FOUR

Breakfast: 1/4 cup orange juice
1/4 cup granola with
1/3 cup skim milk

	1 sl. whole wheat toast with
	1 tsp. margarine
Lunch:	Health Protein Salad—
	1 cup assorted vegies
	1 cup lettuce, bite-size
	1/2 cup chick peas
	1/2 cup cottage cheese, uncreamed
	1 tbsp. each, chopped walnuts, sesame
	seeds, raisins
	1 tbsp. low-calorie bleu cheese dressing
	1 dried prune
Dinner:	Zucchini Parmesan (bake until bubbly)—
	2 cups zucchini, sliced thin, stir-fried
	2 oz. part-skim mozzar. cheese, sliced thin
	1-1/2 cups tomato sauce
	assorted seasonings to taste
	1 slice French bread baked with
	1 tsp. margarine and
	dash garlic powder
	tossed salad with low-calorie dressing
Snack:	1 sm. apple, wedged
	1-1/2 oz. part-skim cheese, cubed

DAY FIVE

Breakfast:	1/2 cup grapefruit sections
	2 sl. French toast (whole wheat) with
	1/4 cup warmed applesauce, unsweetened
Lunch:	Peanut Butter Broil (broil until bubbly)—
	2 sl. cracked wheat bread spread with
	2 tsp. peanut butter
	1/2 banana, sliced
	1 tsp. dried unsweetened coconut
	Blender Shake—
	1 cup skim milk
	1 tsp. honey
	3 dates, chopped
	crushed ice

Dinner:	4 oz. broiled halibut
	5" ear corn on the cob
	1 sm. baked potato with
	1 tbsp. low-cal (imitation) sour cream
	tossed salad with low-cal dressing
Snack:	Cracker melt (broil until bubbly)—
	4 whole rye crackers with
	1 tsp. mustard
	1½ oz. part-skim mozzarella cheese, shredded
	sprouts

DAY SIX

Breakfast:	1/4 canteloupe, 5" dia. filled with
	1/2 cup cottage cheese, uncreamed
	1/4 cup pineapple chunks, unsweetened
	2 tsp. slivered almonds
	1 sl. oatmeal toast with
	1 tsp. margarine
Lunch:	6 oysters on the half shell with
	2 tbsp. cocktail sauce
	2 whole wheat crackers
	3/4 cup yogurt with
	1/2 cup fresh strawberries
Dinner:	3 oz. lean hamburger patty on
	1 whole wheat English muffin with
	lettuce, tomato, onion
	1/2 cup Harvard beets
Snack:	1 cup skim milk
	1 sm. bran muffin

DAY SEVEN

Breakfast:	1/2 grapefruit
	1 egg, scrambled on
	1/2 whole wheat English muffin broiled w/
	1/2 oz. part-skim mozzarella cheese
Lunch:	Vegie Dip (mix and chill)—
	1 cup low-fat yogurt

1/2 cup cottage cheese, uncreamed
3 tbsp. chopped tomato, onion, pepper
Assorted raw vegetable dippers
1 sm. apple baked with
1 tsp. honey and
1 tbsp. chopped walnuts

Dinner: 3 oz. roast veal
1 sm. baked potato with
1 tbsp. low-cal (imitation) sour cream
1/2 cup asparagus
tossed salad with low-calorie dressing

Snack: 4 cups popcorn sprinkled with
4 tbsp. grated parmesan cheese

DAY EIGHT

Breakfast: 1 sm. nectarine
1 cup puffed rice cereal with
1/2 cup skim milk sprinkled with
1 tbsp. each—wheat germ, chopped
walnuts, slivered almonds

Lunch: Eggplant Pocket (bake in foil)—
1 mini whole wheat pita pocket stuffed
with
1 cup sliced eggplant cooked in 1 cup
tomato sauce
1 oz. part-skim mozzarella cheese, sliced thin

Dinner: Fruit Salad Plate—
1/2 cup honey dew melon
1/2 cup strawberries
1/2 cup seedless grapes
1 sm. orange, peeled and sectioned
1/4 sm. banana, sliced
1/4 cup pineapple chunks, unsweetened
1/4 cup cherries
3/4 cup cottage cheese, uncreamed,
sprinkled with 1 tsp. each: wheat germ,
raisins, dried unsweetened coconut

| | 1 tbsp. vanilla low-fat yogurt (as dressing) |
| Snack: | 1 sm. slice carrot cake |

DAY NINE

Breakfast:	1 sm. orange
	1/4 cup Grape Nuts cereal with
	1/3 cup skim milk and
	1/4 cup blueberries
Lunch:	Chef's Salad—
	1 cup lettuce, bite-size
	1 cup assorted vegies
	1 oz. cooked chicken, sliced
	1 oz. part-skim cheese, sliced
	1 egg, hard-boiled, wedged
	sprouts
	1 tbsp. low-calorie French dressing
	1 slice rye bread with
	1 tsp. margarine
Dinner:	Vegetable bake (broil until bubbly)—
	1 cup assorted vegetables, steamed
	3/4 cup brown rice, cooked
	1 oz. part-skim mozzarella cheese
	1 tbsp. each: grated parmesan cheese,
	wheat germ, slivered almonds
	assorted seasonings to taste
	tossed salad with low-cal dressing
Snack:	1 cup skim milk
	2 fig cookies

DAY TEN

Breakfast:	1/2 cup orange juice
	1 egg, poached on
	1/2 pumpernickel bagel broiled with
	1/2 oz. part-skim mozzarella cheese
Lunch:	1 whole wheat English muffin broiled with
	1 oz. part-skim mozzarella cheese and
	sliced tomato-mushroom-pepper

	1 sm. fresh pear
Dinner:	3-1/2 oz. dry white wine
	4 oz. baked chicken
	1 small baked potato with
	1 tsp. margarine
	1/2 cup baby carrots, steamed
	tossed salad with low-calorie dressing
Snack:	Blender Shake—
	1 cup skim milk
	1 tbsp. honey
	1/2 sm. banana, sliced
	crushed ice

DAY ELEVEN

Breakfast:	1 grapefruit
	3 sm. buckwheat pancakes
	1 tbsp. maple syrup
Lunch:	1 cup vegetable soup with
	1 whole wheat breadstick
	1 cup low-fat yogurt with
	1 cup assorted sliced fruit sprinkled with
	2 graham crackers, crumbled
Dinner:	2 tortillas (bean and cheese)
	tossed salad with low-cal dressing
Snack:	5 celery stalks stuffed with
	1 tbsp. peanut butter or
	1-1/2 oz. part-skim cheese, softened

DAY TWELVE

Breakfast:	1 sm. tangerine
	1/2 cup hot oatmeal with
	1/4 cup skim milk and
	1 tbsp. each: wheat germ, chopped
	walnuts, slivered almonds
Lunch:	2 sl. commercial pizza
	1/2 cup fruit cocktail, unsweetened
Dinner:	4 oz. baked haddock

31

1/2 cup Spanish rice
1 sm. whole wheat roll
tossed salad with low-cal dressing

Snack: 1 cup low-fat yogurt with
1/2 cup pineapple chunks, unsweetened &
1 ginger snap, crushed

DAY THIRTEEN

Breakfast: 1/2 cup orange juice
Bagel Broil (broil until bubbly)—
1/2 pumpernickel bagel spread with
1/2 cup cottage cheese, uncreamed
1/4 cup applesauce, unsweetened
dash cinnamon

Lunch: Antipasto—
1 cup lettuce, bite-size
1/2 cup assorted veggies
1 sm. artichoke heart
2 oz. part-skim cheese, sliced
2 sm. black olives
1 tbsp. low-calorie Italian dressing
1 sl. Italian bread with
1 tsp. margarine

Dinner: 3/4 cup macaroni and cheese
1/2 cup broccoli
tossed salad with low-cal dressing

Snack: Blender Shake—
1 cup skim milk
2 tsp. honey
1/2 cup blueberries
crushed ice

DAY FOURTEEN

Breakfast: 1/4 cup fruit salad, unsweetened
1 egg omelet with

	sliced onions, peppers, tomato
	1 sm. bran muffin
Lunch:	Vegetable-gelatin mold with
	1/2 cup cottage cheese, uncreamed
	3 whole rye crackers
	1/2 cup frozen low-fat yogurt
Dinner:	3 oz. roast beef
	1 sm. baked potato with
	1 tbsp. low-cal (imitation) sour cream
	1/2 cup French-style green beans
	tossed salad with low-calorie dressing
	1/2 cup cherries
Snack:	1 sm. pear baked with
	1 tbsp. honey and
	1 tbsp. slivered almonds

DAY FIFTEEN

Breakfast:	1/2 cup pineapple juice
	1/4 cup granola with
	1/3 cup skim milk and
	1/2 sm. banana, sliced
Lunch:	1 whole wheat bagel broiled with
	1-1/2 oz. part-skim mozzarella cheese and
	sliced tomato
	1 cup fresh strawberries with
	1 tbsp. vanilla low-fat yogurt
Dinner:	4 oz. broiled scallops
	1/2 cup mashed potato
	1/3 cup corn
	1 cup coleslaw
Snack:	1 cup skim milk
	3 ginger snaps

DAY SIXTEEN

Breakfast:	1/2 cup grapefruit juice
	1 cup puffed wheat cereal with

Breakfast: 1/2 cup skim milk sprinkled with
1 tbsp. each: wheat germ, chopped
walnuts, slivered almonds

Lunch: Spinach Salad—
1/3 lb. fresh spinach, bite-size
1/2 cup assorted vegies
4 lg. mushrooms, halved
1 egg, hard-boiled, wedges
1 tbsp. imitation bacon bits
1 tbsp. low-calorie Italian dressing
1 sm. fresh pear

Dinner: 3-1/2 oz. chicken breast, baked
1/2 cup cauliflower
1 sm. whole wheat popover
tossed salad with low-cal dressing

Snack: 1 cup skim milk
2 fig cookies

DAY SEVENTEEN

Breakfast: 1/2 cup tangerine sections
1 egg, soft-boiled with
1 whole wheat English muffin

Lunch: Tuna Pocket (bake in foil)—
1 mini whole wheat pita pocket stuffed with
1/2 cup tuna fish
2 tsp. low-cal mayonnaise
3 tbsp. chopped celery-pepper-carrot
1 oz. part-skim mozzarella cheese
1 sm. fresh peach

Dinner: 4 oz. broiled calves' liver with
1/2 cup sliced onions, broiled
1/2 cup brown rice
tossed salad with low-cal dressing

Snack: 1/4 cup raisins with
1/8 cup unsalted peanuts

34

DAY EIGHTEEN

Breakfast: 1/4 cup orange juice
1 biscuit shredded wheat with
1/2 cup skim milk
1 sl. whole wheat toast with
1 tsp. peanut butter

Lunch: Egg Salad Plate—
1 cup lettuce, bite-size
1/2 cup assorted vegies
1/4 cup cottage cheese, uncreamed
1 egg, hard-boiled, chopped, mixed with
2 tsp. low-cal mayonnaise and
1 tbsp. pickle relish
1 tbsp. low-cal bleu cheese dressing
2 whole wheat bread sticks

Dinner: 3 oz. roast lamb
1/2 cup noodles
1/3 cup peas
tossed salad with low-cal dressing

Snack: 1 pear, sliced
1 oz. part-skim cheese, cubed

DAY NINETEEN

Breakfast: 1/2 cup grapefruit sections
1/2 cup hot wheat cereal with
1/4 cup skim milk and
1 tbsp. each: wheat germ, chopped
walnuts, slivered almonds

Lunch: Peanut Butter 'n Date Broil (broil until bubbly)—
2 sl. cracked wheat bread spread with
2 tsp. peanut butter
2 dates, chopped
Blender Shake—
1 cup skim milk
1 tbsp. honey

1/2 sm. banana, sliced
crushed ice

Dinner: 4 oz. broiled swordfish
5" ear corn on the cob
1 sm. baked potato with
1 tbsp. low-cal (imitation) sour cream
Tossed salad with low-cal dressing

Snack: Cracker Melt (broil until bubbly)—
4 whole rye crackers
1 tsp. mustard
1-1/2 oz. part-skim mozzarella cheese, shredde
sprouts

DAY TWENTY

Breakfast: 1/2 grapefruit
1 egg, scrambled on
1/2 whole wheat English muffin, broiled w/
1/2 oz. part-skim mozzarella cheese

Lunch: Vegie Dip (mix and chill)—
1 cup low-fat yogurt
1/2 cup cottage cheese, uncreamed
3 tbsp. chopped tomato-onion-pepper
assorted raw vegetables dippers
1 sm. banana broiled with
1 tbsp. honey

Dinner: 3-1/2 oz. dry red wine
3 oz. roast veal
1/2 cup noodles
1/2 cup spinach
tossed salad with low-cal dressing

Snack: 1 cup skim milk
2 graham crackers

DAY TWENTY-ONE

Breakfast: 1/4 canteloupe, 5" dia., filled with
1/2 cup cottage cheese, uncreamed
1/4 cup pineapple chunks, unsweetened

2 tsp. slivered almonds
1 sl. oatmeal toast with
1 tsp. margarine

Lunch: 3-1/2 oz. dry white wine
Seafood Salad—
1 cup lettuce, bite-size
1/2 cup assorted vegies
6 lg. shrimp
1/2 cup crabmeat
sprouts
1 tbsp. low-cal Russian dressing
4 whole rye crackers

Dinner: 1 cup stir-fried Chinese vegetables on
1/2 cup steamed rice
1 sm. egg roll
tossed salad with
1 oz. part-skim cheese and
1 tbsp. low-cal bleu cheese dressing

Snack: 1 cup low-fat yogurt with
1 cup assorted sliced fruit sprinkled with
2 graham crackers, crumbled

DAY TWENTY-TWO

Breakfast: 1 sm. nectarine
1 cup puffed rice cereal with
1/2 cup skim milk sprinkled with
1 tbsp. each: wheat germ, chopped
walnuts, unprocessed bran

Lunch: Ham 'n Cheese Pocket Bake (bake in foil)
1 mini whole wheat pita pocket stuffed with
1-1/2 oz. boiled ham
1-1/2 oz. part-skim cheese
A tsp. mustard
lettuce, sprouts
1 cup skim milk

Dinner: Fruit Salad Plate—
1/2 cup honeydew melon

1/2 cup strawberries
1/2 cup seedless grapes
1 sm. orange, peeled and sectioned
1/4 sm. banana, sliced
1/4 cup pineapple chunks, unsweetened
1/4 cup cherries
3/4 cup cottage cheese sprinkled with
1 tsp. each: wheat germ, raisins, dried
unsweetened coconut
1 tbsp. vanilla low-fat yogurt (as dressing)

Snack: 1 sm. slice carrot cake

DAY TWENTY-THREE

Breakfast: 1 sm. orange
1/4 cup granola with
1/3 cup skim milk and
1/4 cup fresh blueberries

Lunch: Chef's Salad—
1 cup lettuce, bite-size
1 cup assorted vegies
1 oz. cooked chicken, sliced
1 oz. part-skim cheese, sliced
1 egg, hard boiled, wedges
sprouts
1 tbsp. low-calorie French dressing
1 sl. rye bread with
1 tsp. margarine

Dinner: 4 oz. meatloaf, lean
1 sm. parsley-boiled potato with
1 tsp. margarine
1/2 cup stewed tomatoes
tossed salad with low-cal dressing

Snack: 1 cup skim milk
1 sm. corn muffin

DAY TWENTY-FOUR

Breakfast: 1/2 cup orange juice

            1 egg, hard-boiled
            1/2 sesame bagel with
            2 tsp. peanut butter
Lunch: 1 whole wheat English muffin broiled with
            1-1/2 oz. part-skim cheese and
            sliced tomato, mushrooms, onions
            1 fresh pear
Dinner: 3-1/2 oz. dry white wine
            4 oz. broiled chicken
            1/2 cup asparagus
            1 sm. whole wheat popover
            tossed salad with low-calorie dressing
Snack: Blender Shake—
            1 cup skim milk
            1 tsp. honey
            1 cup sliced apricots, unsweetened
            crushed ice

DAY TWENTY-FIVE

Breakfast: 1/2 grapefruit
            3 sm. buckwheat pancakes with
            1 tbsp. maple syrup
Lunch: 1 cup gazpacho with
            1 whole wheat breadstick
            1 cup low-fat yogurt with
            1 cup assorted sliced fruit and
            2 graham crackers, crumbled
Dinner: 2 Enchilladas (cheese)
            tossed salad with low-cal dressing
Snack: 1 cup skim milk
            1 sm. bran muffin

DAY TWENTY-SIX

Breakfast: 1 sm. tangerine
            1/2 cup hot oatmeal with
            1/4 cup skim milk sprinkled with
            1 tbsp. each: wheat germ, chopped

walnuts, slivered almonds
Lunch: 2 sl. commercial pizza
1/2 cup fruit cocktail, unsweetened
Dinner: 4 oz. poached salmon
1/4 cup rice pilaf
1/2 cup Harvard beets
1/2 cup coleslaw
Snack: 12 oz. "light" beer
10 pretzels (3-ring)

DAY TWENTY-SEVEN

Breakfast: 1/2 cup orange juice
Bagel Broil (broil until bubbly)—
1/2 poppyseed bagel spread with
1/2 cup cottage cheese, uncreamed
1/4 cup applesauce, unsweetened
dash cinnamon
Lunch: Antipasto—
1 cup lettuce, bite-size
1/2 cup assorted vegies
1 sm. artichoke heart
2 oz. part-skim cheese, sliced
2 sm. black olives
1 tbsp. low-calorie Italian dressing
1 sl. Italian bread with
1 tsp. margarine
Dinner: 4 oz. broiled lobster
5" ear corn on the cob
1 sm. baked potato
tossed salad with low-cal dressing
Snack: 4 cups popcorn sprinkled with
4 tbsp. grated parmesan cheese

DAY TWENTY-EIGHT

Breakfast: 1/4 cup fruit salad, unsweetened
1 egg omelet with
sliced onions, peppers, tomatoes

	1 sm. corn muffin
Lunch:	Vegetable-gelatin mold with
	1/2 cup cottage cheese, uncreamed
	3 whole rye crackers
	1/2 cup low-fat frozen yogurt
Dinner:	Shishkabob—
	3 oz. lean lamb, cubed
	3 sm. onions
	3 cherry tomatoes
	3 1" cubes green pepper
	1/2 cup brown rice with
	1 tbsp. slivered almonds
	tossed salad with low-cal dressing
Snack:	1 sm. apple, sliced
	1-1/2 oz. part-skim cheese, chunks

DAY TWENTY-NINE

Breakfast:	1/2 grapefruit
	1 sm. waffle with
	1 tbsp. maple syrup
Lunch:	1/2 sesame bagel
	1/2 poppyseed bagel
	1/2 pumpernickel bagel
	1-1/2 tbsp. cream cheese
	2 fresh plums
Dinner:	I cup spaghetti with
	1 cup tomato sauce and
	2 tbsp. grated parmesan cheese
	1 sl. Italian bread broiled with
	1 tsp. margarine and
	dash garlic powder
	tossed salad with low-cal dressing
Snack:	1 cup skim milk
	2 fig cookies

DAY THIRTY

| Breakfast: | 1/10 casaba melon, 7-3/4" long |

1 biscuit shredded wheat with
1/2 cup skim milk and
1/4 sm. banana, sliced

Lunch: Ham 'n Cheese Pocket Bake (bake in foil)
1 mini whole wheat pita pocket stuffed w/
1-1/2 oz. boiled ham and
1-1/2 oz. part-skim cheese with
1 tsp. mustard
lettuce, sprouts
1 cup skim milk

Dinner: 4 oz. roast turkey
1/2 sm. baked sweet potato
1/8 cup stuffing
1 tbsp. cranberry sauce
1/2 cup green beans
tossed salad with low-cal dressing

Snack: 6 oz. "light" beer
1 sl. conventional pizza

ADDITIONAL NOTES:

a. All fruits and juices should be canned, fresh, or frozen without added sugar.
b. If MENU PLAN indicates "fresh", but fruit is out of season, substitute canned or frozen without added sugar.
c. All vegetables should be canned, fresh or frozen without added seasonings.
d. Cook vegetables rapidly in little water to retain nutrients; try steaming, stir-frying, wok cookery.
e. Eat fruits and vegetables with seeds and skin for added nutritional benefits.
f. Breads, cereals, pastas should be 100% whole grain (e.g. 100% whole wheat).
g. Freeze bagels, breads, English muffins, and rolls; defrost as needed.
h. Choose low-fat dairy products as much as possible.

i. Eggs should be eaten no more than 3 times per week; egg substitute can replace eggs—make sure substitute is a low sodium-no cholesterol variety.

j. Margarine should be tub-style; check label to ensure that the first ingredient is a *liquid* vegetable oil.

k. Canned fish should be water-packed, low-sodium varieties.

l. All meats should be lean and trimmed of all visible fat; bake, boil, broil and roast meats without added fats.

m. All poultry should be lean and eaten without the skin; bake, boil, broil and roast poultry without added fats.

n. Do not fry foods.

o. Peanut butter should be an old-fashioned variety, without added fats or salt.

p. Salad dressings should contain less than 25 calories per tablespoon.

r. Prepare popcorn without added oils or salt; hot air poppers (which do not require the addition of oil) are now available.

s. Occasional sweets or alcoholic beverages may help prevent psychological deprivation and thereby aid in diet adherence.

t. If you want to avoid all sweets and/or alcoholic beverages, use the LISTING and PLANNING COUNTERS to substitute calorically equivalent foods or beverages.

u. Quench your thirst with club soda, black tea or coffee, mineral water, or diet soft drinks; garnish with slices of citrus fruits.

NOTE:

Most foods in the MENU PLAN are low in fat and sodium (salt) in order to promote overall good health in addition to weight loss. Occasional foods containing relatively high contents of calories (or cholesterol and/or sodium) have been included in the MENU PLAN in order to boost dieting morale and prevent rapid diet drop-out.

DINING OUT DO'S and DONT'S

Just because you are on a diet, you do not have to give up the social and psychological pleasures provided by restaurant dining. You do not have to depress yourself with daily brown bag lunches, nor avoid dinner parties and cocktail hours. You can still remain on THE JOY OF BEING THIN DIET PLAN when dining out—at friends' homes, in local cafeterias or in popular restaurants. Try to choose similar selections from your day's MENU; whenever this is impossible, keep in mind the following concepts in order to make low-calorie selections.

DO'S	DONT'S
Appetizers:	
Fresh fruit juices	Fried vegetables
Fresh fruits	Cream soups or chowders
Fruit salad, unsweetened	Chips
Fresh vegetables	Dips
*Vegetable juices	Caviar
*Bouillon or consomme	
Seafood cocktails	

DO'S	DONT'S
Salads:	
Green tossed	Mayonnaise-based salads
Spinach salad	Potato salad
Chef's with lean meats and cheese	Egg salad
Clear vegetable molds	Creamy cole slaw
*Seafood salads	Chef's with fatty meats and cheeses

NOTE: Bring your own low-cal dressings, use vinegar and lemon, or control portions by requesting that dressings be served on-the-side; avoid creamy and cheesy dressings.

DO'S	DONT'S
Breads:	
Whole grain breads	Cheese breads
French or Italian breads	Garlic breads
Pita bread	Submarine rolls
Popovers	Butter rolls
Rolls	Croissants
Bagels	Sweet rolls
English muffins	Breadsticks, salted
Muffins, corn or bran	Crackers, salted
Breadsticks, unsalted	
Crackers, unsalted	
Biscuits	

NOTE: Whole grain products (100% whole) are preferable choices.

DO'S	DONT'S
Meats:	
Lean, trimmed cuts-baked	Breaded, fried cuts
boiled, broiled, roasted	Gravies, potpies, stews
without added fats	Sauces (barbecue, cheese,
	cream, soy, white,
	Worcestershire)

DO'S	DONT'S
Poultry:	
Chicken or turkey,	Goose, duck
skin removed—	
baked, boiled, broiled,	Breaded, fried cuts
roasted without added	Sauces (barbecue, cheese,
fats	cream, soy, white,
	Worcestershire)

DO'S	DONT'S
Fish:	
Any baked, boiled, broiled, poached prepared with minimal use of margarine	Breaded, fried, frozen fillets
*Shellfish	

DO'S	DONT'S
Vegetables:	
Any, plain	Buttered, creamed, fried, seasoned

DO'S	DONT'S
Desserts:	
Angelfood cake	Rich sweets-cake, candy, doughnuts, ice cream, pastries, pies, puddings, etc.
Frozen Fruit ices	
Fruit desserts	
Frozen low-fat yogurt	

DO'S	DONT'S
Beverages:	
Fresh fruit juices	Whole milk
Skim milk	Shakes, eggnog
Coffee, tea	Cream, creamers
Club soda	Sweetened alcoholic drinks
Mineral water	Liqueurs
"Light" beers	
Dry wines	
*Fresh vegetable juices	

DO'S	DONT'S
Extras:	
Lemon juice	Mayonnaise
Vinegar	Sour cream
Herbs, spices	Bacon bits
Cottage cheese, uncreamed	Sweet pickles

Yogurt, low-fat
*Dill pickles

ADDITIONAL NOTES:
   Read menues carefully to avoid selections described as:
       buttered, buttery, butter sauce
       creamed, creamy, cream sauce
       fried, French fried, pan-fried, crispy
       au gratin, escalloped, parmesan
       a la king, bernaise, hollandaise
       casserole, hash, potpie, stew
       all-you-can-eat
       *marinated, pickled, sauteed, smoked

   Remember, the key to successful dining out habits is to follow THE JOY OF BEING THIN DIET PLAN. When this is not possible, choose your foods carefully and eat them in moderation. It may prove wiser NOT to do, than to OVERdo!

*These items should be used in moderation since they are often quite high in sodium (salt).

PERSONAL WEIGHT CHART
   Record your weight once a week on the chart provided on the following page. Then plot your weight on the graph so that yo can visualize your progress more easily.

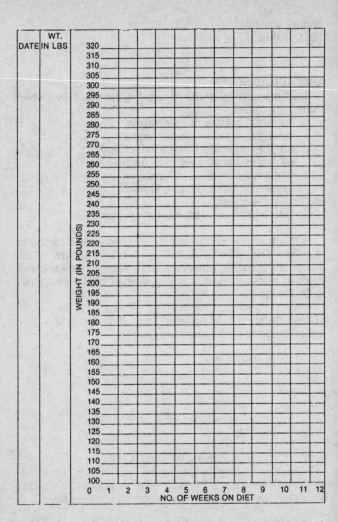

DATE	WT. IN LBS

WEIGHT (IN POUNDS)

320
315
310
305
300
295
290
285
280
275
270
265
260
255
250
245
240
235
230
225
220
215
210
205
200
195
190
185
180
175
170
165
160
155
150
145
140
135
130
125
120
115
110
105
100

0 1 2 3 4 5 6 7 8 9 10 11 12

NO. OF WEEKS ON DIET

HOW TO USE THE FOOD VALUE COUNTERS

To make your dieting a lot simpler, use the information provided in the following food value counters. Whenever you eat—or plan on eating—you can use these counters to determine the approximate amounts per serving of: *CALORIES, FAT,* and *SODIUM.*

The food values provided in these counters were adapted from the latest figures given by the United States Department of Agriculture. Remember, however, that these values are only *estimates!* Variability in size, season, storage and preparation, plus inaccuracies in computations and determinations must be taken into account. Think of it this way:

You have eaten an apple. Using the LISTING COUNTER or the PLANNING COUNTER, you determined the calorie content to be 61 calories. But was that apple *exactly* 2-1/2 inches in diameter? Was it a sweet, ripe variety or a sour type of apple? Was it fresh off the tree in your yard, or did you purchase it several days ago at the local supermarket? And did you eat *every bit* of the edible fruit? And if the apple was eaten as Apple Brown Betty, the specific recipe would have to be considered. After all, your homemade Apple Brown Betty is certainly different from that served in restaurants, and from your friends' recipes.

Manufacturers are constantly altering food products. Food lables can usually provide the most current information on calorie and nutrient contents. This can prove to be especially helpful with those products not included in the food value counters. And if portion sizes given in the counters differ from actual portion sizes eaten, estimates can be made using the COMMON MEASUREMENTS CONVERSION TABLE In the APPENDIX. A METRIC CONVERSION TABLE is also included in the APPENDIX.

Obviously, exact food values are impossible for you to

determine, and impractical for you to be concerned over. The approximate food values given in these counters, however, can be of great assistance in determination of your average daily intake of: CALORIES, FAT, and SODIUM.

The LISTING COUNTER provides the approximate amounts of CALORIES, FAT, and SODIUM in common servings of typical foods. The foods are listed in alphabetical order.

The food value counters can also assist you in planning your meals in advance. Use the PLANNING COUNTER to devise menus for well-balanced, nutritious meals and snacks. The approximate amounts of CALORIES, FAT, and SODIUM in common foods are listed under several headings:

BREAKFAST FOOD SELECTIONS
LUNCH and DINNER FOOD SELECTIONS
SNACK SELECTIONS

One serving of each item in these sections contains no more than: 150 CALORIES, 150 mg. of SODIUM, and minimal (if any) FAT.

The BEVERAGE SELECTIONS section lists a variety of nutritious liquids. One serving of each beverage contains no more than: 120 CALORIES, 150 mg. of SODIUM, and minimal (if any) FAT.

A special counter is also included which provides the food values for the PROTEIN FOOD SELCTIONS. Some of these foods are not as low in CALORIES, SODIUM and/or FAT as the items included in the other 4 sections, but one serving of each provides generous amounts of protein with no more than: 200 CALORIES, 200 mg. of SODIUM, and moderate FAT.

So, good luck! Hopefully, these food value counters can provide the assistance you need for planning, following, and enjoying your diet.

KEY:

The following abbreviations are used in the counters:

cals - calories
pro - protein
fat - fat
carb - carbohydrate
tsp. - teaspoon
tbsp. - tablespoon
oz. - ounce
lb. - pound
sm - small
med. - medium
mini. - miniature
sl. - slice
pkg. - package
dia. - diameter
sq. - square
" - inch
cu. in. - cubic inch

ADDITIONAL NOTES:

The food values given in the counters reflect the following:
- All flour is enriched.
- All cornmeal is degermed, enriched.
- All canned fruits and vegetables are drained.
- A measured cup is spooned in, rather than packed.
- Unless otherwise noted, products are medium sized.
- "Homemade" items were made according to the U.S. Department of Agriculture's own standardized recipes.

FOOD	AMOUNT	CALS	FAT (g.)

A

FOOD	AMOUNT	CALS	FAT (g.)
Almonds:			
dried, shelled, chopped	1 tbsp.	48	4.3
roasted, salted	1 cup	984	90.6
shelled, slivered	1 cup	688	62.3
Almond meal, partially defatted	1 oz.	116	5.2
Amaranth leaves, fresh	1 lb.	163	2.3
Anchovies, canned, 4" long	5	35	2.1
Apple Brown Betty	1 cup	325	7.5
Apple butter	1 tbsp.	33	.1
Apples:			
dehydrated, uncooked	1 cup	353	2.0
dried, rings	1 cup	234	1.4
fresh, whole, 3" dia.	1	96	1.0
fresh, whole, 2½" dia.	1	61	.6
juice, canned or bottled	1 cup	117	t
Applesauce:			
canned, sweetened	1 cup	232	.3
canned, unsweetened	1 cup	100	.5
Apricots:			
canned, sweetened	1 cup	222	.3
canned, unsweetened	1 cup	93	.2
dehydrated, uncooked	1 cup	332	1.0
dried, uncooked	1 cup	338	.7
fresh, halves	1 cup	79	.3
fresh, whole	3	55	.2
nectar, canned or bottled (40% fruit)	1 cup	143	.3

FOOD	AMOUNT	CALS	FAT (g.)
Artichokes:			
French or globe, cooked	1 bud	16	.2
Jerusalem, pared, cooked	4 oz.	75	.2
Asparagus:			
canned, spears	1 cup	51	1.0
fresh, cuts	1 cup	35	.3
fresh, cuts, cooked	1 cup	29	.3
fresh, spears, cooked	1 cup	36	.4
frozen, cuts, cooked	1 cup	44	.4
frozen, spears, cooked	1 cup	40	.4
Avocados:			
California, 3⅛" dia.	1	369	36.7
Florida, 3⅝" dia.	1	389	33.4

B

FOOD	AMOUNT	CALS	FAT (g.)
Bacon:			
Canadian, cooked	1 sl.	58	3.
cured, cooked	1 sl.	43	3.
Baking powder:			
phosphate	1 tsp.	5	
sodium aluminum sulfate	1 tsp.	3	
special low sodium	1 tsp.	7	
tartrate	1 tsp.	2	
Bamboo shoots, fresh	1 cup	41	
Bananas:			
baking (see Plantain)			
dehydrated, flakes	1 cup	340	
fresh, 9¾" long	1	116	
fresh, 8¾" long	1	101	
fresh, 7¾" long	1	81	

FOOD	AMOUNT	CALS	FAT (g.)
fresh, mashed	1 cup	191	.5
fresh, red, 7¼" long	1	118	.3
fresh, sliced	1 cup	128	.3
Barbeque sauce	1 cup	228	17.3
Barley, pearled:			
light, uncooked	1 cup	698	2.0
pot or Scotch, uncooked	1 cup	696	2.2
Bass, fresh oven-fried	4 oz.	224	9.6
Bean curd (see Soybeans)			
Beans:			
dry, pinto, uncooked	1 cup	663	2.3
dry, red kidney, cooked	1 cup	218	.9
dry, white, Great Northern, cooked	1 cup	212	1.1
dry, white, Navy (pea), cooked	1 cup	224	1.1
dry, white, with meat and molasses	1 cup	383	12.0
dry, white, with meat and tomato sauce	1 cup	311	6.6
dry, white, with meatless tomato sauce	1 cup	306	1.3
green or snap, canned	1 cup	32	.3
green or snap, fresh	1 cup	35	.2
green or snap, fresh, cooked	1 cup	31	.3
green or snap, frozen, cooked	1 cup	34	.1
French style, canned	1 cup	31	.3
French style, frozen, cooked	1 cup	34	.1
lima, canned	1 cup	163	.5

FOOD	AMOUNT	CALS	FAT (g.)
lima, fresh, cooked	1 cup	189	.9
lima, frozen, cooked ("baby")	1 cup	212	.4
lima, frozen, cooked ("fordhook")	1 cup	168	.2
sprouts, mung	1 cup	37	.2
sprouts, mung, cooked	1 cup	35	.3
yellow or wax, canned	1 cup	32	.4
yellow or wax, fresh	1 cup	30	.2
yellow or wax, fresh, cooked	1 cup	28	.3
yellow or wax, frozen, cooked	1 cup	36	.1
Bean Sprouts (see Beans, Soybeans)			
Beans and franks, canned	1 cup	367	18.1
Beechnuts, shelled	1 oz.	161	14.3
Beef, lean, trimmed, cooked:			
boneless chuck for stew	1 cup	300	13.3
chuck, rib roast or steak, choice grade	3 oz.	212	11.8
chuck, rib roast or steak, good grade	3 oz.	186	8.7
chuck roast or steak, choice grade	3 oz.	164	6.0
chuck roast or steak, good grade	3 oz.	152	4.4
flank steak (London broil)	3 oz.	167	6.2
ground, 10% fat	3 oz.	186	9.6
ground, 21% fat	3 oz.	259	18.3
loin, clubsteak	4 oz.	515	46.1
loin, porterhouse steak	4 oz.	254	11.9

FOOD	AMOUNT	CALS	FAT (g.)
loin, t-bone steak	4 oz.	253	11.7
plate beef	4 oz.	226	8.7
rib roast	3 oz.	205	11.4
round steak	3 oz.	161	5.2
rump roast, choice grade	3 oz.	177	7.9
rump roast, good grade	3 oz.	162	6.0
sirloin, double-bone	3 oz.	184	8.1
sirloin, hipbone	3 oz.	204	10.6
sirloin, wedge- and round-bone	3 oz.	176	6.5
Beef and vegetable stew, canned	1 cup	194	7.6
Beef, corned:			
canned, cooked	4 oz.	245	13.6
canned, hash	1 cup	398	24.9
fresh, cooked	4 oz.	422	34.5
Beef, dried:			
chipped, creamed	1 cup	377	25.2
chipped, uncooked	1 oz.	58	1.8
Beef pot pie, homemade, 9" dia.	1/3 pie	517	30.5
Beer (see Beverages)			
Beet greens, cooked	1 cup	26	.3
Beets:			
canned, diced or sliced	1 cup	63	.2
canned, whole, small	1 cup	59	.2
fresh, diced or sliced, cooked	1 cup	54	.2
fresh, whole, 2" dia., cooked	2	32	.1
Harvard	1 cup	80	t
pickled	1 cup	80	t

FOOD	AMOUNT	CALS	FAT (g.)
Beverages, alcoholic:			
ale (7% alcohol)	12 oz.	168	0
beer (4.5% alcohol)	12 oz.	151	0
beer "light"	12 oz.	96	t
gin, rum, vodka, whiskey			
(86 proof)	1½ oz.	105	t
(100 proof)	1½ oz.	124	t
wine, dessert			
(18.8% alcohol)	3½ oz.	141	0
table (12% alcohol)	3½ oz.	87	0
Beverages, carbonated*:			
club soda,			
unsweetened	12 oz.	0	0
cola	12 oz.	144	0
cream soda	12 oz.	160	0
fruit flavored sodas	12 oz.	171	0
ginger ale	12 oz.	113	0
root beer	12 oz.	152	0
special "diet" sodas	12 oz.	0-12	0
Tom Collins mixer	12 oz.	171	0
tonic water	12 oz.	113	0
Biscuit, baking powder:			
from mix, 2" dia.	1	91	2.6
homemade, 2" dia.	1	103	4.8
Blackberries:			
canned, sweetened	1 cup	233	1.5
canned, unsweetened	1 cup	98	1.5
*fresh	1 cup	84	1.3
**frozen, sweetened	1 cup	60	.4
**frozen, unsweetened	1 cup	137	.4

*depends on sodium content of water supply at bottling plant
*includes dewberries, boysenberries, youngberries
**includes boysenberries

FOOD	AMOUNT	CALS	FAT (g.)
juice, canned, unsweetened	1 cup	91	1.5
Blackeye peas (see Cowpeas)			
Blood pudding (see Sausage)			
Blueberries:			
fresh	1 cup	90	.7
frozen, sweetened	1 cup	242	.7
frozen, unsweetened	1 cup	91	.8
Bluefish:			
fresh, baked with margarine	4 oz.	185	5.9
fried fillet, 8⅛" long	1 fillet	400	19.1
Bockwurst (see Sausage)			
Bologna (see Cold Cuts)			
Boston brown bread, canned, ½" thick	1 sl.	95	.6
Bouillon, instant:			
cube	1	5	.1
powder	1 tsp.	2	.1
Boysenberries (see Blackberries)			
Bran (see Cereals)			
Braunschweiger (see Sausage)			
Brazil nuts:			
shelled, large	1 cup	916	93.7
shelled, large	6	185	19.0
Bread:			
cracked wheat	1 sl.	66	.6
French (2½"x2"x½")	1 sl.	44	.5
Italian (4½"x3¼"x¾")	1 sl.	83	.2
pumpernickel	1 sl.	79	.4
pumpernickel, party-size	1 sl.	17	.1
raisin	1 sl.	66	.7

FOOD	AMOUNT	CALS	FAT (g.)
rye	1 sl.	61	.3
rye, party-size	1 sl.	17	.1
white, firm-crumb, regular	1 sl.	63	.9
white, firm-crub, thin	1 sl.	41	.6
white, soft-crumb	1 sl.	76	.9
whole wheat, firm-crumb	1 sl.	61	.8
whole wheat, soft-crumb	1 sl.	67	.7
Bread crumbs:			
dry, grated	1 cup	392	4.6
soft, cubed	1 cup	81	1.0
Bread pudding, with raisins	1 cup	496	16.2
Bread sticks, 4½" long	1	38	.3
Bread stuffing:			
mix, dry, crumbs	1 cup	260	2.7
prepared, crumbly	1 cup	501	30.5
prepared, moist	1 cup	416	25.6
Breakfast cereals (see Cereals)			
Broadbeans, dry, raw	1 oz.	96	.5
Broccoli:			
fresh, cuts, cooked	1 cup	40	.5
fresh, stalks	1 med.	47	.5
frozen, chopped, cooked	1 cup	48	.6
frozen, stalks, cooked	8 med.	65	.5
Brownies (see Cookies)			
Brussels sprouts:			
fresh, cooked	1 cup	56	.6
frozen, cooked	1 cup	51	.3
Buckwheat (see Flour)			

FOOD	AMOUNT	CALS	FAT (g.)
Bulgur:			
canned, seasoned	1 cup	246	4.5
canned, unseasoned	1 cup	227	.9
dry, from club wheat	1 cup	628	2.5
dry, from hard red wheat	1 cup	602	2.6
dry, from winter wheat	1 cup	553	1.9
Butter:			
regular type	1 stick	812	91.9
regular type	1 tbsp.	102	11.5
regular type	1 pat	36	4.1
whipped type	1 tbsp.	67	7.6
Buttermilk (see Milk)			
Butternuts, shelled	1 oz.	178	17.3

C

FOOD	AMOUNT	CALS	FAT (g.)
Cabbage:			
Chinese, chopped	1 cup	11	.1
red, chopped	1 cup	28	.2
savoy, sliced	1 cup	17	.1
spoon (pakchoy) chopped, cooked	1 cup	24	.3
white, chopped	1 cup	22	.2
white, wedges, cooked	1 cup	31	.3
Cabbage salad (see Coleslaw)			
Cake, from mix:			
Angelfood, cube	1 cu. in.	6	t
9¾" dia.	2½" arc	137	.1
chocolate, white icing, 9" dia.	1¾" arc.	232	5.8
coffeecake, 7¾" x 5⅝"	1/16 cake	232	6.9

FOOD	AMOUNT	CALS	FAT (g.)
cupcake, uniced, 2½" dia.	1	88	3.0
cupcake, chocolate icing, 2½" dia.	1	129	4.5
devil's food, chocolate icing, 9" dia.	1¾" arc	234	8.5
gingerbread, 8¼" dia.	2¾" sq.	174	4.3
marble, white icing, 9" dia.	1¾" arc.	215	5.7
spice, caramel icing, 9" dia.	1¾" arc.	271	8.3
white, chocolate icing 9" dia.	1¾" arc.	249	7.6
yellow, chocolate icing 9" dia.	1¾" arc	233	7.8
Cakes, frozen:			
devil's food, choc. icing, 7½"x1¾"	4" sq.	323	15.0
Cake, homemade:			
Boston cream pie, 8" dia.	2⅛" arc.	208	6.5
cottage pudding, 2"x4"	1 sl.	186	6.1
fruitcake, dark 7" tube	2/3" arc	163	6.6
fruitcake, light, 7" tube	2/3" arc	167	7.1
pound, 3½x3x½	1 sl.	142	8.9
sponge, 9¾" tube	2½" arc.	131	2.5
Cake icings:			
from mix, chocolate	1 tbsp.	79	2.8
homemade, carmel	1 tbsp.	77	1.4
homemade, chocolate	1 tbsp.	65	2.4
uncooked white	1 tbsp.	75	1.3

FOOD	AMOUNT	CALS	FAT (g.)
Candied fruits (see individual kinds)			
Candy:			
butterscotch	1 oz.	113	1.0
candycorn	1 cup	728	4.0
caramels, plain or chocolate	1 oz.	113	2.9
caramels, with nuts	1 oz.	121	4.6
chocolate, bittersweet	1 oz.	135	11.3
chocolate, semi-sweet	1 oz.	144	10.1
chocolate, sweet	1 oz.	150	10.0
chocolate, milk, plain	1 oz.	147	9.2
chocolate, milk, with almonds	1 oz.	151	10.1
chocolate, milk, with peanuts	1 oz.	154	10.8
chocolate coated-almonds	1 oz.	161	12.4
chocolate coated-coconut	1 oz.	124	5.0
chocolate coated-mints, 2½" dia.	1 oz.	144	3.7
chocolate coated-fudge, caramel, peanuts	1 oz.	123	5.1
chocolate coated-honeycomb, peanut butter	1 oz.	131	5.5
chocolate coated-noughat, caramel	1 oz.	118	3.9
chocolate coated-peanuts	1 oz.	159	11.7
chocolate coated-raisins	1 oz.	120	4.8
chocolate coated-vanilla creams	1 oz.	123	4.8

FOOD	AMOUNT	CALS	FAT (g)
fudge, chocolate	1 cu. in.	84	2.6
fudge, chocolate with nuts	1 cu. in.	89	3.7
fudge, vanilla	1 cu. in.	84	2.3
gumdrops	1 oz.	98	.2
hard	1 oz.	109	.3
jellybeans	10	104	.1
marshmallows, large 1⅛" dia.	1	23	
marshmallows, mini ½" dia.	1 cup	147	
mints, round, 1½" dia.	1	32	.2
mints, square, ⅝"x⅝"	1 cup	400	2.2
peanut bars	1 oz.	146	9.1
peanut brittle	1 oz.	119	2.9
sugar coated almonds	1 oz.	129	5.3
sugar coated chocolate disks	1 oz.	132	5.6
Cantaloupe, fresh:			
5" dia.	1/2	82	.3
diced	1 cup	48	.2
Capicola (see Cold cuts)			
Carob flour (see Flour)			
Carrots:			
canned, diced	1 cup	44	.4
canned, sliced	1 cup	47	.5
fresh, 7" long	1	30	.1
fresh, grated	1 cup	46	.2
fresh, diced, cooked	1 cup	45	.2
fresh, sliced, cooked	1 cup	48	.5
Casaba melon, fresh:			
7¾" long	1/10	38	
diced or balls	1 cup	46	
Cashew nuts, roasted	1 cup	785	64.0

FOOD	AMOUNT	CALS	FAT (g.)
Catsup, tomato, bottled	1 tbsp.	16	.1
Cauliflower:			
fresh, whole buds	1 cup	27	.2
fresh, cooked	1 cup	28	.3
frozen, cooked	1 cup	32	.4
Caviar, sturgeon:			
granular	1 tbsp.	42	2.4
pressed	1 tbsp.	54	2.8
Celery, fresh:			
8″ long	1 stalk	7	t
diced	1 cup	20	.1
diced, cooked	1 cup	21	.2
Cereal:			
bran, added sugar	1 cup	144	1.8
bran flakes (40% bran)	1 cup	106	.6
bran flakes with raisins	1 cup	144	.7
corn flakes	1 cup	97	.1
corn flakes, sugar-coated	1 cup	154	.1
corn, puffed, presweetened	1 cup	114	.1
corn, puffed, presweetened, cocoa-flavor	1 cup	117	.7
corn, puffed, presweetened, fruit-flavor	1 cup	119	.8
farina, instant, cooked	1 cup	135	.2
farina, quick, cooked	1 cup	105	.2
farina, regular, cooked	1 cup	103	.2
oat flakes, maple-flavored, cooked	1 cup	166	1.9
oat granules, maple-flavored, cooked	1 cup	147	1.5
oatmeal or rolled oats,			

FOOD	AMOUNT	CALS	FAT (g.)
dry	1 cup	312	5.9
oatmeal or rolled oats, cooked	1 cup	132	2.4
oats, shredded, sweetened	1 cup	171	.9
rice, granulated, cooked	1 cup	123	†
rice, oven-popped	1 cup	117	.1
rice, oven-popped, presweetened	1 cup	175	.3
rice, puffed	1 cup	60	.1
rice, puffed, presweetened	1 cup	140	1.4
rice, puffed, presweetened, cocoa-flavor	1 cup	140	1.4
wheat flakes	1 cup	106	.5
wheat germ	1 tbsp.	23	.7
wheat, puffed	1 cup	54	.2
wheat, puffed, presweetened	1 cup	132	.7
wheat, shredded	1 biscuit	89	.5
wheat, shredded, spoon size	1 cup	177	1.0
wheat, whole meal, cooked	1 cup	110	.7
wheat with malted barley, instant, cooked	1 cup	196	.7
wheat with malted barley, quick, cooked	1 cup	159	.7
Cervelat (see Sausage)			
Chard, Swiss, fresh, cooked	1 cup	26	.3
Cheese:			
American, processed	1 oz.	106	8.9

FOOD	AMOUNT	CALS	FAT (g.)
American, processed	1 cu. in.	66	5.5
American, processed, shredded	1 cup	418	2.1
blue or roquefort	1 cup	497	41.2
blue or roquefort	1 oz.	104	8.6
brick	1 oz.	105	8.6
brick	1 cu. in.	64	5.1
brie	1 oz.	95	7.9
camembert, domestic	1 oz.	85	6.9
cheddar, domestic	1 oz.	114	9.4
cheddar, domestic	1 cu. in.	68	5.5
cheddar, domestic, shredded	1 cup	455	37.5
colby	1 oz.	112	9.1
colby	1 cu. in.	68	5.5
cottage, creamed,	1 cup	217	9.5
cottage, low-fat (2%)	1 cup	203	4.4
cottage, uncreamed	1 cup	123	.6
cream	1 tbsp.	52	5.3
cream, whipped	1 tbsp.	37	3.8
edam	1 oz.	101	7.9
feta	1 oz.	75	6.0
gouda	1 oz.	101	7.8
limburger	1 oz.	93	7.7
mozzarella, part-skim	1 oz.	72	4.5
neufchatel	1 oz.	74	6.6
parmesan	1 oz.	111	7.3
parmesan, grated	1 cup	467	30.8
parmesan, grated	1 tbsp.	23	1.5
provalone	1 oz.	100	7.6
ricotta, part-skim	1 cup	340	19.5
Swiss, domestic	1 oz.	107	7.8
Swiss, domestic	1 cu. in.	56	4.1

FOOD	AMOUNT	CALS	FAT (g.)
Swiss, processed	1 oz.	95	7.1
Swiss, processed	1 cu. in.	60	4.5
Swiss, domestic	1 oz.	107	7.8
Swiss, domestic	1 cu. in.	56	4.1
Swiss, processed	1 oz.	95	7.1
Swiss, processed	1 cu. in.	60	4.5
Cheese food, American, processed	1 tbsp.	45	3.4
Cheese spread, American	1 tbsp.	40	3.0
Cheese straws, 5" long	1	27	1.8
Cherimoya, fresh, 5" dia.	1/4	115	.5
Cherries:			
candied	10	119	.1
sour, canned, unsweetened	1 cup	105	.5
sour, fresh, whole, (pitted)	1 cup	90	.5
sweet, canned, sweetened	1 cup	208	.5
sweet, canned, unsweetened	1 cup	119	.5
sweet, fresh, whole (pitted)	1 cup	102	.4
Chestnuts:			
in shell	10	141	1.1
shelled	1 cup	310	2.4
Chewing gum, sweetened	1 stick	6	0
Chicken, lean, trimmed, cooked (no skin):			
broiler	4 oz.	154	4.3
fryer, dark meat, fried	4 oz.	250	10.6
fryer, light meat, fried	4 oz.	224	6.9
hen or cocks,			

FOOD	AMOUNT	CALS	FAT (g.)
chopped	1 cup	291	12.5
roaster, dark meat	4 oz.	209	7.4
roaster, light meat	4 oz.	207	5.6
roaster, light meat, chopped	1 cup	255	6.9
Chicken a la king, homemade	1 cup	468	34.3
Chicken, canned, meat only	1 cup	406	24.0
Chicken pot pie, homemade, 9" dia.	1/3 pie	545	31.3
Chickpeas (Garbanzos), raw	1 cup	720	9.6
Chicory, fresh, chopped	1 cup	14	.1
Chili con carne, with beans, canned	1 cup	339	15.6
Chili sauce, tomato, bottled	1 tbsp.	16	t
Chives, fresh, chopped	1 tbsp.	1	t
Chocolate, baking: bitter	1 oz.	143	15.0
semi-sweet, morsels or chips	1 cup	862	60.7
Chocolate, bittersweet or sweet (see Candy)			
Chocolate candy (see Candy)			
Chocolate milk (see Milk)			
Chocolate syrup: thin type	2 tbsp.	92	.8
fudge topping	2 tbsp.	124	5.1
Chop suey, with meat, homemade	1 cup	300	17.0
Chow mein, with meat, homemade	1 cup	255	10.0
Cider (see Apple, juice)			

FOOD	AMOUNT	CALS	FAT (g.)
Citron, candied .... 1 oz.	89	.1
Clams:			
canned, chopped or			
minced .... 1 cup	157	4.0
fresh, hard or round,			
raw .... 1 pint	363	4.1
fresh, soft, raw .... 1 pint	372	8.6
juice, bottled .... 1 cup	46	.2
Cocoa:			
beverage powder .... 1 oz.	98	.6
medium fat powder .... 1 tbsp.	14	1.0
medium fat powder, with			
alkali .... 1 tbsp.	14	1.0
Coconut:			
dried, unsweetened .... 1 oz.	188	18.4
fresh .... 2" sq.	156	15.9
fresh, shredded .... 1 cup	277	28.2
Coconut liquid:			
cream .... 1 tbsp.	50	4.8
milk .... 1 cup	605	59.8
water .... 1 cup	53	.5
Cod:			
canned, flaked .... 1 cup	119	.4
dehydrated, shredded .... 1 cup	158	1.2
dried, salted .... 1 oz.	37	.2
fresh, broiled with			
margarine .... 4 oz.	192	6.0
Coffee, prepared, plain .... 1 cup	2	t
Cola (see Beverages)			
Cold cuts:			
bologna, all meat .... 1 oz.	79	6.5
bologna, with binders .... 1 oz.	74	5.8
braunschweiger (smoked			
liverwurst) .... 1 oz.	90	7.8

FOOD	AMOUNT	CALS	FAT (g.)
capicola	1 oz.	141	13.0
deviled ham, canned	1 tbsp.	46	4.2
liverwurst, unsmoked	1 oz.	87	7.2
luncheon meat (see Luncheon meats)			
mortadella	1 oz.	89	7.1
salami	1 oz.	128	10.8
Coleslaw, commercial:			
with boiled dressing	1 cup	114	8.8
with mayonnaise	1 cup	173	16.8
Collards:			
fresh, cooked	1 cup	63	1.3
frozen, chopped, cooked	1 cup	51	.7
Cookies:			
animal crackers	10	112	2.4
brownie, from mix, 1¾" sq.	1	86	4.0
brownie, frozen, iced, 1½"x1¾"	1	103	5.0
brownie, homemade, with nuts, 1¾" sq.	1	97	6.3
butter thins, 2" dia.	1	23	.9
chocolate chips, commercial 2¼" dia.	1	50	2.2
chocolate chip, homemade, 2 1/3" dia.	1	51	3.0
coconut bars, 3 x 1¼"	1	45	2.2
fig bars, 1⅝" sq.	1	50	.8
gingersnaps, 2" dia.	1	29	.6
graham crackers, chocolate coated	2" sq.	62	3.1
graham crackers, plain	2"sq.	28	.7
graham crackers, sugar-honey	2" sq.	29	.8

FOOD	AMOUNT	CALS	FAT (g.)
ladyfingers, 3¼" long	1	40	.9
macaroons, 2¾" dia.	1	90	4.4
marshmallow, chocolate-coated, 2⅛" dia.	1	53	1.7
marshmallow, coconut-coated, 2⅛" dia.	1	74	2.4
molasses, 3⅝" dia.	1	137	3.4
oatmeal, with raisins, 2⅝" dia.	1	59	2.0
peanut sandwich cookies, 1¾" dia.	1	58	2.4
peanut sugar wafers, 1¾" x 1⅜"	1	33	1.3
plain, 1⅝" dia.	1	28	1.4
raisin, 2¼"x2"	1	54	.8
sandwich-type, oval	1	74	3.4
sandwich-type, round	1	50	2.3
sandwich-type, peanut (see Cookie, peanut)			
shortbread, 1⅝" sq.	1	37	1.7
sugar, homemade, 2¼" dia.	1	36	1.3
sugar wafers, 2½"x¾"	1	17	.7
vanilla wafers, 1¾" dia.	1	19	.6
vanilla wafers, brown edge, 2¾" dia.	1	27	.9
Cookie dough, plain, chilled, baked, 2½" dia.	1	60	3.0
Corn:			
canned, cream style	1 cup	210	1.5
canned, kernels	1 cup	139	1.3
fresh, kernels, cooked	1 cup	137	1.7
fresh, on the cob, cooked	5" ear	70	.8

FOOD	AMOUNT	CALS	FAT (g.)
frozen, kernels, cooked	1 cup	130	.8
frozen, on the cob, cooked	5" ear	118	1.2
Corn bread:			
from mix	2½" sq.	178	5.8
homemade	2½" sq.	186	5.0
Corn cereal (see Cereals)			
Corn flour (see Flour)			
Corn fritters, 2" dia.	1	132	7.5
Corn grits, degermed, cooked	1 cup	125	.2
Cornmeal:			
degermed, cooked	1 cup	120	.5
degermed, dry	1 cup	502	1.7
whole, dry	1 cup	433	4.8
Corn muffins (see Muffins)			
Corn oil (see Oils)			
Corn pone, 9" dia	3½" arc	122	3.2
Corn pudding	1 cup	255	11.5
Cornstarch	1 tbsp.	29	t
Cottonseed oil (see Oils)			
Cottage cheese (see Cheeses)			
Cottage pudding (see Cakes)			
Cowpeas (including blackeye peas)			
canned	1 cup	179	.8
fresh, cooked	1 cup	178	1.3
frozen, cooked	1 cup	221	.7
Crab:			
canned, claw	1 cup	116	2.9
canned, white or king	1 cup	136	3.4
fresh, steamed	1 lb.	422	8.6
fresh, steamed, flaked	1 cup	116	2.4
fresh, steamed, pieces	1 cup	144	2.9

FOOD	AMOUNT	CALS	FAT (g.)
Cracker crumbs:			
butter	1 cup	366	14.2
graham	1 cup	326	8.0
soda	1 cup	307	9.2
Crackers:			
animal (see Cookies)			
butter, round 1⅞" dia.	1	15	.6
cheese, 1" sq.	10	52	2.3
graham (see Cookies)			
rye wafers, 3½"x1⅞"	1	22	t
saltines, 1⅞" sq.	1	12	.3
sandwich-type, cheese-peanut butter, 1⅝" sq.	1	35	1.7
soda, 1⅞" sq.	1	12	.4
soda, biscuit, 2⅜" x 2⅛"	1	22	.7
soda, soup or oyster	1 cup	198	5.9
wheat thins	4	55	3.1
zwieback, 3½"x1½	1	30	.6
Cranberries, fresh, whole	1 cup	44	.7
Cranberry juice cocktail, sweetened	1 cup	164	.3
Cranberry-orange relish	1 cup	490	1.1
Cranberry sauce, canned, sweetened	1 cup	404	.6
Cream:			
half and half	1 tbsp.	20	1.7
light or table	1 tbsp.	29	2.9
sour	1 tbsp.	26	2.5
whipped (pressurized)	1 cup	154	13.3
whipped, unsweetened	1 cup	419	44.8
whipping, heavy	1 tbsp.	52	5.6
Cream puff, custard filling, 3½" dia.	1	303	18.1
Cream substitute,			

FOOD	AMOUNT	CALS	FAT (g.)
non-dairy	1 tbsp.	20	1.5
Cress, garden, cooked	1 cup	31	.8
Cress, water (see Watercress)			
Cucumbers:			
peeled, 6⅜" long	1	22	.2
peeled, sliced	1 cup	20	.1
pickled (see Pickles)			
Cusk, steamed	1 oz.	30	.2
Custard, baked	1 cup	305	14.6
Custard, frozen (see Ice cream)			

D

FOOD	AMOUNT	CALS	FAT (g.)
Dandelion greens, cooked	1 cup	35	.6
Danish pastry, commercial			
4½" dia.	1	274	15.3
Dates, pitted:			
chopped	1 cup	488	.9
whole	10	219	.4
Deviled ham (see Cold cuts)			
Dewberries (see Blackberries)			
Doughnuts:			
cake-type, plain 3⅝" dia.	1	227	10.8
yeast leavened, 3¾" dia.	1	176	11.3

E

FOOD	AMOUNT	CALS	FAT (g.)
Eclair, custard filled, choc. frosted,			
5" long	1	239	13.6
Egg, chicken, large:			
fried	1	99	7.9
hard cooked	1	82	5.8
omelet or scrambled	1	111	8.3

FOOD	AMOUNT	CALS	FAT (g.)
poached	1	82	5.8
raw, white	1	17	t
raw, whole	1	82	5.8
raw, yolk	1	59	5.2
Eggnog	1 cup	342	19.0
Eggplant, fresh, cooked	1 cup	38	.4
Egg substitute	1 cup	384	26.7
Endive, fresh, chopped	1 cup	10	.1
Escarole (see Endive)			

F

FOOD	AMOUNT	CALS	FAT (g.)
Farina (see Cereals)			
Fat, vegetable			
shortening	1 tbsp.	111	12.5
Figs:			
canned, sweetened	1 cup	218	.5
canned, unsweetened	1 cup	119	.5
dried	1	55	.2
fresh, 2¼" dia.	1	40	.2
Filberts (hazelnuts):			
in shell	10	87	8.6
shelled, chopped	1 tbsp.	44	4.4
shelled, whole	1 cup	856	84.2
Fish (see individual kinds)			
Fish cakes, frozen, breaded, fried, 3" dia.	1	103	4.8
Fish flakes, canned	1 cup	183	1.0
Fish sticks, frozen, breaded, cooked	1 oz. stick	50	2.5
Flounder, fresh, baked with margarine	4 oz.	228	9.2
Flour:			
all purpose, sifted	1 cup	419	1.2

FOOD	AMOUNT	CALS	FAT (g.)
bread, sifted	1 cup	420	1.3
buckwheat, dark, sifted	1 cup	326	2.5
buckwheat, light, sifted	1 cup	340	1.2
cake or pastry, sifted	1 cup	349	.8
carob	1 cup	495	2.0
corn	1 cup	431	3.0
gluten (45%)	1 cup	510	2.6
rye, dark, unsifted	1 cup	419	3.3
rye, light, unsifted	1 cup	364	1.0
soybean, defatted	1 cup	326	.9
wheat, whole	1 cup	400	2.4
Frankfurters:			
all meat smoked, 4¾" long	1	124	10.7
all meat, unsmoked, 5" long	1	133	11.5
canned, 4⅞" long	1	106	8.7
with binders, 5" long	1	112	9.3
Frostings (see Cake icings)			
Frozen custard (see Ice cream)			
Fruit (see individual kinds)			
Fruit cocktail:			
canned, sweetened	1 cup	194	.3
canned, unsweetened	1 cup	91	.2
Fruit salad:			
canned, sweetened	1 cup	191	.3
canned, unsweetened	1 cup	86	.2

G

Garbanzos (see Chick peas)			
Garlic, raw	1 clove	4	t

FOOD	AMOUNT	CALS	FAT (g.)
Gelatin:			
dry 1/4 oz. envelope 1		23	t
dessert, prepared .... 1 cup		142	0
Gin (see Beverages)			
Ginger ale (see Beverages)			
Gingerbread (see Cake)			
Ginger root:			
candied .... 1 oz.		96	0.1
fresh .... 1 lb.		207	4.2
Gluten flour (see Flour)			
Goat milk (see Milk)			
Goose, domesticated,			
cooked .... 3 oz.		198	8.3
Gooseberries, fresh .... 1 cup		59	.3
Granadilla (passion fruit),			
fresh 1		16	.1
Grapefruit:			
canned, sweetened .... 1 cup		178	.3
canned, unsweetened .... 1 cup		73	.2
fresh, 3-9/16" dia. 1/2		40	.1
fresh, sections .... 1 cup		82	.2
juice, canned,			
sweetened .... 1 cup		133	.3
juice, canned,			
unsweetened .... 1 cup		101	.2
juice, fresh .... 1 cup		96	.2
juice, frozen,			
sweetened .... 1 cup		117	.2
juice, frozen,			
unsweetened .... 1 cup		101	.2
Grapefruit-orange juice:			
canned, sweetened .... 1 cup		125	.2
canned, unsweetened .... 1 cup		106	.5
frozen, unsweetened .... 1 cup		109	.2

FOOD	AMOUNT	CALS	FAT (g.)
Grapes:			
canned, sweetened	1 cup	197	.3
canned, unsweetened	1 cup	125	.2
fresh, American-type	1 cup	70	1.0
fresh, European-type	1 cup	107	.5
juice, canned	1 cup	167	t
juice, frozen, sweetened	1 cup	133	t
Grape drink (30% grape juice)	1 cup	135	t
Grits (see Corn)			
Groundcherries, fresh	1 cup	74	1.0
Guava, fresh	1 med.	48	t
Gum (see Chewing Gum)			

H

FOOD	AMOUNT	CALS	FAT (g.)
Haddock, fresh, oven-fried	4 oz.	188	7.2
Halibut, fresh, broiled with margarine	4 oz.	192	8.0
Ham (see Pork)			
Hamburger (see Beef)			
Hazelnuts (see Filberts)			
Hash (see Beef, corned)			
Headcheese (see Sausage)			
Heart, lean, cooked, chopped:			
beef	1 cup	273	8.3
calf	1 cup	302	13.2
chicken	1 cup	268	11.5
hog	1 cup	283	10.0
lamb	1 cup	377	20.9
turkey	1 cup	257	8.81

FOOD	AMOUNT	CALS	FAT (g.)
Herring:			
canned, plain, 3½" long 1		221	14.5
canned, tomato sauce,			
4¾" long 1		97	5.8
pickled, 7" long 1		112	7.6
smoked, 7" long 1		137	8.4
Hominy grits (see Corn grits)			
Honey, strained			
or extracted .... 1 tbsp.		64	0
Honeydew melon:			
fresh, 7" long .... 1/10 melon		49	.4
fresh, diced or balls .... 1 cup		56	.5
frozen balls,			
sweetened .... 1 cup		143	.2
Horseradish, prepared .... 1 tbsp.		6	t
Hyacinth-beans, young pods,			
cuts .... 1 cup		32	.3

I

FOOD	AMOUNT	CALS	FAT (g.)
Ice cream			
plain, 10% fat .... 1 cup		269	14.3
plain, 16% fat .... 1 cup		349	23.7
soft serve			
(frozen custard) .... 1 cup		377	22.5
Ice milk:			
plain, 5% fat .... 1 cup		184	5.6
soft serve .... 1 cup		223	4.6
Icings (see Cake icings)			

FOOD	AMOUNT	CALS	FAT (g.)

J

Jams and preserves, all flavors	1 tbsp.	54	t
Jellies, all flavors	1 tbsp.	49	t
Jerusalem artichokes (see Artichokes)			
Juices (see individual kinds)			

K

Kale:			
fresh, cooked	1 cup	43	.8
frozen, cooked	1 cup	40	.7
Kidney, beef, sliced, cooked	1 cup	353	16.8
Kippered herring (see Herring, smoked)			
Knockwurst (see Sausage)			
Kohlrabi, fresh, diced, cooked	1 cup	40	.2
Kumquat, fresh	1 sml.	15	t

L

Ladyfingers (see Cookies)			
Lamb, lean, trimmed, cooked:			
leg	3 oz.	158	6.0
loin chops	4 oz.	213	8.5
rib chops	4 oz.	240	12.0
shoulder	3 oz.	174	8.5
shoulder, diced	1 cup	287	14.0

FOOD	AMOUNT	CALS	FAT (g.)
Lard	1 tbsp.	117	13.0
Leeks (see Onions)			
Lemons:			
fresh, 2⅛" dia.	1	20	.2
juice, canned, unsweetened	1 tbsp.	3	t
juice, fresh	1 tbsp.	4	t
juice, frozen, unsweetened	1 tbsp.	3	t
Lemonade, frozen, sweetened	1 cup	107	t
Lemon peel, candied	1 oz.	90	.1
Lentils, dry, cooked	1 cup	212	t
Lettuce, raw:			
Boston or bibb, large leaf	1 leaf	2	t
Boston or bibb, shredded or chopped	1 cup	8	.1
iceberg, wedge	1/4 head	18	.1
iceberg, shredded or chopped	1 cup	7	.1
looseleaf, shredded or chopped	1 cup	10	.2
romaine, shredded or chopped	1 cup	10	.2
Lima beans (see Beans, lima)			
Limes:			
fresh, 2" dia.	1	19	.1
juice, canned, unsweetened	1 tbsp.	4	t
juice, fresh	1 tbsp.	4	t
Limeade, frozen, sweetened	1 cup	102	t
Liver, cooked:			
beef (fried)	3 oz.	195	9.0

FOOD	AMOUNT	CALS	FAT (g.)
calf (fried)	3 oz.	222	11.2
chicken	4 oz.	187	5.0
chicken, chopped	1 cup	231	6.2
hog (fried)	3 oz.	205	9.8
lamb	4 oz.	296	14.1
turkey, chopped	1 cup	244	6.7
Liver paste (see Pate de foie gras)			
Liverwurst (see Sausage)			
Lobster fresh or canned:			
cooked	1 lb.	431	6.8
cooked, chopped	1 cup	138	2.2
Lobster Newberg	1 cup	485	26.5
Lobster paste, canned	1 tsp.	13	.7
Loganberries, fresh	1 cup	89	.9
Loquats, fresh	10	59	.2
Luncheon meat, canned or packaged:			
boiled ham	1 oz.	66	4.8
pork, chopped	1 oz.	83	7.1
Lychees, fresh	10	58	.3

M

FOOD	AMOUNT	CALS	FAT (g.)
Macaroni, cooked:			
cold	1 cup	117	.4
hot	1 cup	155	.6
Macaroni and cheese:			
canned	1 cup	228	9.6
homemade	1 cup	430	22.2
Mackerel:			
Atlantic, fresh, broiled with margarine	4 oz.	268	16.0
Pacific, canned	3 oz.	153	8.5
salted	1 oz.	86	7.1

FOOD	AMOUNT	CALS	FAT (g.)
Malt, dry	1 oz.	104	.5
Malt extract, dried	1 oz.	104	t
Mandarin oranges (see Tangerines)			
Mangos, fresh:			
diced	1 cup	109	.7
whole	1	152	.9
Margarine:			
regular	1 stick	816	91.9
regular or soft	1 tbsp.	102	11.5
regular	1 pat	36	4.1
whipped	1 tbsp.	68	7.6
Marmalade, citrus	1 tbsp.	51	t
Matai (see Waterchestnuts)			
Mayonnaise (see Salad dressings)			
Meat (see individual kinds)			
Melons (see individual kinds)			
Milk, cow's:			
buttermilk	1 cup	99	2.2
chocolate, hot	1 cup	218	9.1
chocolate-flavored, low-fat	1 cup	179	5.0
chocolate-flavored, whole	1 cup	208	8.5
condensed, sweetened	1 cup	982	26.6
dried, non-fat, instant	1 cup	244	.5
evaporated, canned	1 cup	338	19.0
low-fat, 2%	1 cup	121	4.7
skim	1 cup	86	.4
whole	1 cup	157	8.9
Milk, goat's, whole	1 cup	168	10.1
Milk, malted, powder	1 oz.	116	2.4
Mixed vegetables (see Vegetables, mixed)			

FOOD	AMOUNT	CALS	FAT (g.)
Molasses, cane:			
light	1 tbsp.	50	t
blackshop	1 tbsp.	43	t
Mortadella (see Cold cuts)			
Muffins:			
from mix, corn 2⅜" dia.	1	130	4.2
homemade, blueberry, 2⅜" dia.	1	112	3.7
homemade, bran, 2⅜" dia.	1	104	3.9
homemade, corn, 2⅜" dia.	1	126	4.0
homemade, plain, 3" dia.	1	118	4.0
Mushrooms:			
canned, chopped or sliced	1 cup	42	—
fresh, chopped or sliced	1 cup	20	.2
Muskmelons (see individual kinds)			
Mustard greens:			
fresh, cooked	1 cup	32	.6
frozen, chopped, cooked	1 cup	30	.6
Mustard spinach, fresh, cooked	1 cup	29	.4
Mustard, prepared:			
brown	1 tsp.	5	.3
yellow	1 tsp.	4	.2
Mussels:			
canned	4 oz.	129	—
fresh	4 oz.	108	—

N

Nectarines, fresh, 2½" dia.	1	88	t

FOOD	AMOUNT	CALS	FAT (g.)
Noodles:			
chowmein, canned	1 cup	220	10.6
egg, cooked	1 cup	200	2.4
Nuts (see individual kinds)			

O

FOOD	AMOUNT	CALS	FAT (g.)
Oats, oatmeal (see Cereal)			
Oil:			
cooking or salad*	1 tbsp.	120	13.6
olive	1 tbsp.	119	13.5
peanut	1 tbsp.	119	13.5
Okra:			
fresh, sliced	1 cup	36	.3
fresh, sliced, cooked	1 cup	46	.5
frozen, sliced, cooked	1 cup	70	.2
Oleomargarine (see Margarine)			
Olive oil (see Oil)			
Olives, pickled, canned or bottled:			
green, large, ¾" dia.	10	45	4.9
green, small, ⅝" dia.	10	33	3.6
ripe, ascolano, ¾" dia.	10	61	6.5
ripe, ascolano, sliced	1 cup	174	18.6
Olives, ripe:			
manzanillo, ¾" dia.	10	61	6.5
manzanillo, sliced	1 cup	174	18.6
mission, ¾" dia.	10	87	9.5
mission, sliced	1 cup	248	27.1
salt 'n oil (Greek style)	10	65	6.9
sevillano, 1" dia.	10	95	9.7

*corn, cottonseed, safflower, sesame, soybean oils, and
soybean-cottonseed oil blend

FOOD	AMOUNT	CALS	FAT (g.)
Onions:			
dehydrated	1 tbsp.	18	t
green, bulb and top, chopped	1 tbsp.	2	t
green, bulb and white, chopped	1 tbsp.	3	t
green, tops only, chopped (scallions)	1 tbsp.	2	t
mature, chopped	1 cup	65	.2
mature, whole or sliced, cooked	1 cup	61	.2
Oranges, fresh:			
Florida, 2⅝" dia.	1	66	.3
naval, 2⅞" dia.	1	71	.1
Valencia, 2⅝" dia.	1	62	.4
sections	1 cup	88	.4
Orange Juice:			
canned, sweetened	1 cup	130	.5
canned, unsweetened	1 cup	120	.5
fresh	1 cup	112	.5
frozen, unsweetened	1 cup	114	.7
Orange-cranberry relish (see cranberry-orange relish)			
Orange-grapefruit juice (see grapefruit-orange juice)			
Orange peel, candied	1 oz.	90	.1
Oysters, raw, meat only:			
Eastern, 13-19 med.	1 cup	158	4.3
Pacific and Western, 4-6 med.	1 cup	218	5.3
Oysters, fried, 2-3 med.	1 oz.	68	3.9
Oyster stew, homemade	1 cup	233	15.4

P

FOOD	AMOUNT	CALS	FAT (g.)
Pancakes:			
from mix, buckwheat, 6" dia. 1		146	6.6
from mix, buckwheat, 4" dia. 1		54	2.5
from mix, plain & buttermilk, 6" dia. 1		164	5.3
from mix, plain & buttermilk, 4" dia. 1		61	2.0
homemade, 6" dia. 1		169	5.1
homemade, 4" dia. 1		62	1.9
Papaws, fresh, 2" dia. 1		83	.9
Papayas:			
fresh, 3½" dia. 1		119	.3
fresh, cubed .... 1 cup		55	.1
Parsley, fresh:			
chopped .... 1 tbsp.		2	t
whole sprigs 10		4	.1
Parsnips, cooked:			
diced .... 1 cup		102	.8
mashed .... 1 cup		139	1.1
whole, 6" long 1		23	.2
Passion fruit (see Granadilla)			
Pastina, egg, dry .... 1 cup		651	7.0
Pastry shell (see Pie crust)			
Pate de foie gras, canned .... 1 tbsp.		60	5.7
Peaches:			
canned, sweetened .... 1 cup		200	.3
canned, unsweetened .... 1 cup		76	.2
dehydrated, uncooked .... 1 cup		340	.9

FOOD	AMOUNT	CALS	FAT (g.)
dried halves, uncooked	10 med.	341	.9
fresh, 2½" dia.	1	38	.1
fresh, diced	1 cup	70	.2
frozen, sweetened, sliced	1 cup	220	.3
nectar, canned (40% fruit)	1 cup	120	t
Peanut butter, commercial	1 tbsp.	94	8.1
Peanuts, roasted:			
in shell, jumbo	10	105	8.8
shelled, chopped	1 tbsp.	52	4.4
shelled, salted, chopped or whole	1 cup	842	71.7
shelled, salted, Spanish	20	53	4.5
shelled, salted Virginia	10	53	4.5
Peanut oil (see Oils)			
Pears:			
canned, sweetened	1 cup	194	.5
canned, unsweetened	1 cup	78	.5
dried halves, uncooked	10	469	3.2
fresh, Bartlett, 2½" dia.	1	100	.7
fresh, Bosc, 2½" dia.	1	86	.6
fresh, D'Anjou, 3" dia.	1	122	.8
fresh, sliced or cubed	1 cup	101	.7
nectar, canned (40% fruit)	1 cup	130	.5
Peas:			
blackeye (see Cowpeas)			
green, canned, early or June	1 cup	150	.7
green, canned, sweet	1 cup	136	.7
green, fresh	1 cup	122	.6

FOOD	AMOUNT	CALS	FAT (g.)
green, fresh, cooked	1 cup	114	.6
green, frozen, cooked	1 cup	109	.5
split, cooked	1 cup	230	.6
Peas and carrots, frozen, cooked	1 cup	85	.5
Pecans:			
in shell, large (64-77/lb.)	10	236	24.5
shelled, chopped	1 tbsp.	52	5.3
shelled, halves	1 cup	742	76.9
Peppers:			
hot, green, canned	1 cup	49	.2
hot, red, canned	1 cup	51	1.5
sweet green, 3" dia.	1 ring	2	t
sweet green, sliced	1 cup	18	.2
sweet green, sliced, cooked	1 cup	24	.3
sweet red, 3" dia.	1 ring	3	t
sweet red, sliced	1 cup	25	.2
Perch:			
fresh, cooked	4 oz.	130	—
ocean (redfish), fresh	4 oz.	100	—
Persimmons, fresh:			
Japanese or kaki, 2½" dia.	1	129	.7
native	1	31	.1
Pickles, cucumber:			
"bread and butter," slices, ¼" thick	2	11	t
dill, slices, ¼" thick	2	1	t
dill, spear, 6" long	1	3	.1
dill, whole, 4" long	1	15	.3
sour, whole, 4" long	1	14	.3
sweet, chopped	1 tbsp.	15	t
sweet, gherkin, 3" long	1	51	.1
sweet, gherkin, midget	1	9	t

FOOD	AMOUNT	CALS	FAT (g.)
sweet, spear, 4½" long	1	29	.1
Pickles, mustard (chow-chow):			
sour	1 tbsp.	70	.2
sweet	1 tbsp.	18	.1
Pickle relish, sweet	1 tbsp.	21	.1
Pie:			
apple, frozen, baked, 8" dia.	4⅛" arc	231	9.1
apple, homemade, 9" dia.	3½" arc	302	13.1
banana custard, homemade, 9" dia.	3½ arc	252	10.6
blackberry, homemade, 9" dia.	3½" arc	287	13.0
blueberry, homemade, 9" dia.	3½" arc	286	12.7
Boston cream (see Cake)			
cherry, frozen, baked, 8" dia.	4⅛" arc	282	11.7
cherry, homemade, 9" dia.	3½" arc	308	13.3
chocolate chiffon, homemade 9" dia.	3½" arc	266	12.4
coconut custard, from mix, 8" dia.	4⅛" arc	270	10.5
coconut custard, frozen, baked, 8" dia.	4⅛" arc	249	12.0
coconut custard, homemade, 9" dia.	3½" arc	268	14.3
custard, homemade, 9" dia.	3½" arc	249	12.7
lemon meringue, homemade, 9" dia.	3⅛" arc	268	10.7

FOOD	AMOUNT	CALS	FAT (g.)
mince, homemade, 9" dia.	3½" arc	320	13.6
peach, homemade, 9" dia.	3½" arc	301	12.6
pecan, homemade, 9" dia.	3½" arc	431	23.6
pineapple, homemade, 9" dia.	3½" arc	299	12.6
pumpkin, homemade, 9" dia.	3½" arc	241	12.8
rhubarb, homemade, 9" dia.	3½" arc	299	12.6
strawberry, homemade, 9" dia.	3½" arc	184	7.3
sweet potato, homemade, 9" dia.	3½" arc	243	12.9
Piecrust or plain pastry:			
baked, 9" dia.	1 shell	900	60.1
from mix, 10 oz. pkg., baked	1 shell	1485	93.1
Pignolias (see Pinenuts)			
Pigs' feet, pickled	2 oz.	113	8.4
Pimentoes, canned, with liquid	2 oz.	15	.3
Pineapple:			
canned, sweetened, cuts*	1 cup	189	.3
canned, sweetened, sliced, 3" dia.	1 ring	43	.1
canned, unsweetened, cuts*	1 cup	96	.2
Pineapple:			
fresh, diced	1 cup	81	.3
fresh, sliced, 3½" dia.	1	44	.2

FOOD	AMOUNT	CALS	FAT (g.)
frozen, sweetened, chunks	1 cup	208	.2
juice, canned, unsweetened	1 cup	138	.3
juice, frozen, unsweetened	1 cup	130	.1
Pineapple, candied	1 oz.	90	.1
Pineapple and grapefruit juice drink, canned (50% fruit juices)	1 cup	135	.1
Pineapple and orange juice drink, canned (40% fruit juice)	1 cup	135	.3
Pinenuts:			
pignolias, shelled	1 oz.	156	13.4
pinons, shelled	1 oz.	180	17.2
Pistachio nuts, shelled	1 oz.	168	15.2
Pitanga, fresh, pitted	1 cup	87	.7
Pizza:			
frozen, baked, 10" dia.	4½" arc	139	4.0
frozen, baked, 5¼" dia.	1 pizza	179	5.2
homemade, 14" diam.	5-1/3" arc	153	5.4
Plantain (baking bananas), fresh, 11" long	1	313	1.1
Plums:			
canned, sweetened	1 cup	214	.3
canned, unsweetened	1 cup	114	.5
fresh, Damson, 1" dia.	10	66	t
fresh, Damson, halves	1 cup	112	t
fresh, Japanese, 2⅛" dia.	1	32	.1
fresh, Japanese, diced	1 cup	79	.3

FOOD	AMOUNT	CALS	FAT (g.)
fresh, prune-type, 1½" dia.	1	21	.1
fresh, prune type, halves	1 cup	124	.3
Poha (see Groundcherries)			
Pokeberry shoots, cooked	1 cup	33	.7
Pollock, fresh creamed	1 cup.	320	14.8
Pomegranate, fresh, 3⅜" dia.	1	97	.5
Popcorn, popped:			
plain	1 cup	23	.3
salt and oil added	1 cup	41	2.0
sugar-coated	1 cup	134	1.2
Popovers, homemade, 4" high	1	90	3.7
Pork, lean, trimmed, cooked:			
ham, cured	3 oz.	159	7.5
ham, cured, canned	4 oz.	214	13.9
ham, fresh	3 oz.	184	8.5
ham, fresh, diced	1 cup	304	14.0
ham, fresh, ground	1 cup	239	11.0
loin chops, fresh	3 oz.	226	13.0
loin roast, fresh	3 oz.	216	12.1
shoulder, Boston butt, cured	3 oz.	207	11.7
shoulder, Boston butt, fresh	3 oz.	207	12.2
shoulder, picnic, cured	3 oz.	179	8.4
shoulder, picnic, fresh	3 oz.	180	8.3
spareribs (with fat)	4 oz.	499	44.1
Pork sausage (see Bacon)			
Potato, sweet:			
baked in skin, 4¾" long	1	161	.6
boiled in skin, 4¾" long	1	172	.6
boiled in skin, mashed	1 cup	291	1.0

FOOD	AMOUNT	CALS	FAT (g.)
candied in syrup, 2½" long	1	176	3.5
canned, chopped	1 cup	216	.4
Potato, white:			
baked in skin, 4¾" long	1	145	.2
boiled, in skin, 2½" dia.	1	104	.1
boiled, peeled, 2½" dia.	1	73	.1
boiled, peeled, diced or sliced	1 cup	101	.2
dehydrated flakes, prepared	1 cup	195	6.7
dehydrated granules, prepared	1 cup	202	7.6
French fried, 2-3½" long	10	137	6.6
French fried, 1-2" long	10	96	4.6
French fried, frozen, oven-heated, 2-3½"	10	110	4.2
French fried, frozen, oven-heated, 1-2"	10	77	2.9
fried	1 cup	456	24.1
hash brown, cooked	1 cup	355	18.1
mashed, with milk	1 cup	137	1.5
scalloped	1 cup	255	9.6
Potato chips	10	114	8.0
Potato salad:			
with cooked salad dressing	1 cup	248	7.0
with mayonnaise and eggs	1 cup	363	23.0
Potato sticks	1 cup	190	12.7
Pretzels:			
logs, 3" long	10	195	2.3
rods, 7½" long	1	55	.6
sticks, 3⅛" long	10	23	.3
sticks, 2¼" long	10	12	.1

FOOD	AMOUNT	CALS	FAT (g.)
twisted, 3-ring	10	117	1.4
twisted, 1-ring	10	78	.9
twisted, Dutch	1	62	.7
twisted, thins	10	234	2.7
Prunes:			
dehydrated, uncooked	1 cup	344	.5
dried, chopped	1 cup	408	1.0
dried, large	1	22	t
dried, medium	1	16	t
juice, canned or bottled	1 cup	197	.3
Prune whip, baked	1 cup	140	.2
Pudding:			
from mix, chocolate	1 cup	322	7.8
from mix, instant, chocolate	1 cup	325	6.5
homemade, chocolate	1 cup	385	12.2
homemade, vanilla	1 cup	283	9.9
Pumpkin, canned	1 cup	81	.7
Pumpkin seeds, hulled	1 cup	774	65.4

Q

Quail, fresh, cooked	4 oz.	190	—
Quince, fresh	4 oz.	65	—

Rabbit, domesticated, cooked, chopped	1 cup	302	14.1
Radishes, fresh:			
large	10	14	.1

FOOD	AMOUNT	CALS	FAT (g.)
sliced	1 cup	20	.1
Raisins, seedless:			
chopped	1 cup	390	.3
whole	1 cup	419	.3
whole	1 tbsp.	26	t
Raspberries:			
fresh, black	1 cup	98	1.9
fresh, red	1 cup	70	.6
frozen, red, sweetened	1 cup	245	.5
Redfish (see Perch)			
Rhubarb:			
fresh, diced	1 cup	20	.1
fresh, sweetened, cooked	1 cup	381	.3
frozen, sweetened, cooked	1 cup	386	.5
Rice, cooked:			
brown, long grain	1 cup	232	1.2
white, long grain	1 cup	223	.2
white, long grain, parboiled	1 cup	186	.2
white, long grain, pre-cooked (instant)	1 cup	180	t
Rice cereal (see Cereal)			
Rice polish	1 cup	278	13.4
Rice pudding, with raisins	1 cup	387	8.2
Rockfish, fresh, cooked	4 oz.	120	2.8
Roe, herring, canned	4 oz.	134	3.2
Rolls and buns, commercial, ready-to-serve:			
cloverleaf or dinner, 2" high	1	83	1.6
frankfurter or hamburger	1	119	2.2

FOOD	AMOUNT	CALS	FAT (g.)
hard roll, 3¾" dia. 1		156	1.6
hoagie or submarine, 11½"			
long 1		392	4.1
Romaine (see Lettuce)			
Root beer (see Beverages)			
Rum (see Beverages)			
Rusk, 3⅜" dia. 1		38	.8
Rutabagas, fresh, cooked:			
cubed .... 1 cup		60	.2
mashed .... 1 cup		84	.2
Rye flour (see Flour)			
Rye wafers (see Crackers)			

S

Safflower oil (see Oils)			
Salad dressings, commercial:			
blue cheese or			
roquefort .... 1 tbsp.		76	7.8
blue cheese or roquefort, low-			
calorie .... 1 tbsp.		12	.9
French .... 1 tbsp.		66	6.2
French, low calorie .... 1 tbsp.		15	.7
Italian .... 1 tbsp.		83	9.0
Italian, low-calorie .... 1 tbsp.		8	.7
mayonnaise .... 1 tbsp.		101	11.2
Russian .... 1 tbsp.		74	7.6
Russian, low-calorie .... 1 tbsp.		23	.7
salad dressing (mayonnaise-			
type) .... 1 tbsp.		65	6.3
salad dressing, low			
calorie .... 1 tbsp.		22	2.0
thousand island .... 1 tbsp.		80	8.0

FOOD	AMOUNT	CALS	FAT (g.)
thousand island, low calorie	1 tbsp.	27	2.1
Salad dressing, homemade, cooked	1 tbsp.	26	1.6
Salad oil (see Oils)			
Salami (see Cold cuts)			
Salmon, canned:			
Atlantic	1 cup	447	26.8
chinook (king)	1 cup	462	30.8
*chum	1 cup	306	11.4
coho (silver)	1 cup	337	15.6
pink (humpback)	1 cup	310	13.0
sockeye (red)	1 cup	376	20.5
Salmon, fresh:			
broiled with margarine	4 oz.	208	8.4
smoked	4 oz.	200	10.4
Salsify, fresh, cubed, cooked	1 cup	94	.8
Salt, table:			
	1 cup	0	0
	1 tbsp.	0	0
	1 tsp.	0	0
Sardines, Atlantic, canned, 3" long	1	24	1.3
Sauces, (see individual kinds)			
Sauerkraut, canned	1 cup	42	.5
Sausage:			
blood (blood pudding)	1 oz.	112	10.5
bockwurst	1 link	172	15.4
brown-and-serve, cooked	1 link	72	6.4
cervelat	1 oz.	128	10.7
country-style	1 oz.	98	8.8
headcheese	1 oz.	76	4.4

FOOD	AMOUNT	CALS	FAT (g.)
knockwurst	1 link	189	15.8
Polish, 5⅜" long	1 link	231	19.6
pork, canned	1 link	46	3.9
pork, fresh, cooked	1 link	62	5.7
scrapple	1 oz.	61	3.9
souse	1 oz.	51	3.8
summer (thuringer cervelat)	1 oz.	87	6.9
Vienna, canned, 2" long	1 link	38	3.2
Scallions (see Onions)			
Scallops:			
bay and sea, fresh, cooked	4 oz.	127	1.4
bay and sea, frozen, breaded, fried, reheated	4 oz.	220	9.5
Scrapple (see Sausage)			
Sesame oil (see Oils)			
Sesame seeds, dry, hulled	1 tbsp.	47	4.3
Shad, fresh, baked	4 oz.	228	12.8
Shallot, bulbs, fresh, chopped	1 tbsp.	7	t
Sherbet, orange	1 cup	270	3.8
Shortbread (see Cookies)			
Shrimp:			
canned (22-76)	1 cup	148	1.4
fresh, meat only 2½" long	10	37	.4
fried	4 oz.	256	12.4
Shrimp paste, canned	1 tsp.	13	.7
Smelt, fresh	7 med.	100	—
Snails, raw, meat only	4 oz.	100	—
Soft drinks (see Beverages)			

FOOD	AMOUNT	CALS	FAT (g.)
Sole, fresh, cooked	4 oz.	90	—
Soup, canned, condensed:			
asparagus, cream of, prepared with milk	1 cup	147	5.9
asparagus, cream of, prepared with water	1 cup	65	1.7
bean with pork, prepared with water	1 cup	355	12.2
beef broth or consomme, prepared with water	1 cup	31	0
beef noodle, prepared with water	1 cup	67	2.6
celery, cream of, prepared with milk	1 cup	169	9.3
celery, cream of, prepared with water	1 cup	86	5.0
chicken, consomme, prepared with water	1 cup	22	t
chicken, cream of, prepared with milk	1 cup	179	10.3
chicken, cream of, prepared with water	1 cup	94	5.8
chicken gumbo, prepared with water	1 cup	55	1.4
chicken noodle, prepared with water	1 cup	62	1.9
chicken vegetable, prepared with water	1 cup	76	2.5
chicken with rice, prepared with water	1 cup	48	1.2
clam chowder (Manhattan type), prepared with water	1 cup	81	2.5
minestrone, prepared with water	1 cup	105	3.4

FOOD	AMOUNT	CALS	FAT (g.)
mushroom, cream of, prepared with milk	1 cup	216	14.2
mushroom, cream of, prepared with water	1 cup	134	9.6
onion, prepared with water	1 cup	65	2.4
pea, green, prepared with water	1 cup	130	2.2
pea, split, prepared with water	1 cup	145	3.2
tomato, prepared with milk	1 cup	173	7.0
tomato, prepared with water	1 cup	88	2.5
turkey noodle, prepared with water	1 cup	79	2.9
vegetable beef, prepared with water	1 cup	78	2.2
vegetable with beef broth, prepared with water	1 cup	78	1.7
vegetarian vegetable, prepared with water	1 cup	78	2.0
Soup, dehydrated, prepared according to package:			
beef noodle	1 cup	67	1.2
chicken noodle	1 cup	53	1.4
chicken with rice	1 cup	48	1.0
onion	1 cup	36	1.2
pea, green	1 cup	123	1.5
Sour cream (see Cream)			
Soursop, raw, pureed	1 cup	146	.7
Souse (see Sausages)			
Soybeans:			
curd (tofu) 2½"x2¾"	1 piece	86	5.0

FOOD	AMOUNT	CALS	FAT (g.)
dry, cooked	1 cup	234	10.3
flour (see Flour)			
oil (see Oil)			
sprouts	1 cup	48	1.5
sprouts, cooked	1 cup	48	1.8
Soy sauce	1 tbsp.	12	.2
Spaghetti:			
canned, in tomato sauce,			
cheese	1 cup	190	1.5
canned, with meatballs and			
sauce	1 cup	258	10.3
plain, cooked,			
"al dente"	1 cup	192	.7
plain, cooked, tender			
stage	1 cup	155	.6
with homemade tomato sauce,			
cheese	1 cup	260	8.8
Spanish rice, homemade	1 cup	213	4.2
Spinach:			
canned	1 cup	49	1.2
fresh, chopped	1 cup	14	.2
fresh, cooked	1 cup	41	.5
frozen, chopped,			
cooked	1 cup	47	.6
frozen, leaf, cooked	1 cup	46	.6
Spot, fresh, baked	4 oz.	336	24.8
Squash, summer, fresh:	1 cup	25	.1
Squash, summer, cooked,			
sliced:			
crookneck or straight-			
neck	1 cup	27	.4
scallop varieties	1 cup	29	.2
zucchini or Italian	1 cup	22	.2
Squash, winter, fresh:			

FOOD	AMOUNT	CALS	FAT (g.)
acorn, baked, 4" diam.	1/2	86	.2
butternut, baked, mashed	1 cup	139	.2
butternut, boiled, mashed	1 cup	100	.2
hubbard, baked, mashed	1 cup	103	.8
hubbard, boiled, diced	1 cup	71	.7
hubbard, boiled, mashed	1 cup	74	.7
Squash, winter, frozen, cooked	1 cup	91	.7
Starch, (see Cornstarch)			
Strawberries:			
fresh, whole	1 cup	55	.7
frozen, sweetened, sliced	1 cup	278	.5
frozen, sweetened, whole	1 cup	235	.5
Sturgeon:			
fresh, cooked	4 oz.	180	6.4
smoked	4 oz.	168	2.0
Succotash, frozen, cooked	1 cup	158	.7
Sugar, beet or cane:			
brown, packed	1 cup	821	0
granulated	1 cup	770	0
granulated	1 tsp.	15	0
granulated	1 packet	23	0
powdered, sifted	1 cup	385	0
powdered, unsifted	1 cup	462	0
Sugar, maple	1 oz.	99	—
Sunflower seeds, hulled	1 cup	812	68.6
Surinam cherry (see Pitanga)			
Sweet potatoes (see Potato, sweet)			

FOOD	AMOUNT	CALS	FAT (g.)
Swiss chard (see Chard, Swiss)			
Sword fish, fresh, broiled with			
margarine	4 oz.	184	6.4
Syrup			
chocolate (see Chocolate syrup)			
corn, light or dark	1 cup	951	0
corn, light or dark	1 tbsp.	59	0
maple	1 tbsp.	50	t
sorghum	1 cup	848	t
sorghum	1 tbsp.	53	t
table blend (cane and			
maple)	1 tbsp.	50	0

T

FOOD	AMOUNT	CALS	FAT (g.)
Tangelo:			
fresh, 2¾" dia.	1	47	.1
juice, fresh	1 cup	101	.2
Tangerine, fresh:			
2½" dia.	1	46	.2
sections	1 cup	90	.4
juice, canned,			
sweetened	1 cup	125	.5
juice, canned,			
unsweetened	1 cup	106	.5
juice, fresh	1 cup	106	.5
juice, frozen,			
unsweetened	1 cup	114	.5
Tapioca:			
dried	1 cup	535	.3
pudding	1 cup	221	8.4
Tartar sauce	1 tbsp.	74	8.1
Thuringer (see Sausage)			

FOOD	AMOUNT	CALS	FAT (g.)
Tilefish, fresh, baked	4 oz.	156	4.0
Tomatoes:			
canned	1 cup	51	.5
fresh, 2-3/5" dia.	1	27	.2
fresh, cooked	1 cup	63	.5
juice, canned or bottled	1 cup	46	.2
juice cocktail, canned or bottled	1 cup	51	.2
Tomato catsup (see Catsup)			
Tomato chili sauce (see Chili sauce)			
Tomato paste, canned	1 cup	215	1.0
Tomato puree, canned	1 lb.	177	.9
Tongue cooked:			
beef	2 oz.	138	9.5
calf	2 oz.	91	3.8
hog	2 oz.	144	9.9
lamb	2 oz.	144	10.3
sheep	2 oz.	183	14.4
Tripe, canned	4 oz.	113	—
Trout, fresh, cooked	4 oz.	225	—
Tuna:			
canned in oil	1 cup	315	13.1
canned in water	4 oz.	144	.9
fresh, cooked	3 oz.	105	—
salad	1 cup	349	21.5
Turkey:			
canned, meat only	1 cup	414	25.6
cooked, chopped	1 cup	266	8.5
cooked, dark meat	3 oz.	173	7.1
cooked, light meat	3 oz.	150	3.3
Turkey giblets, cooked, chopped	1 cup	338	22.3
Turkey pot pie, homemade,			

FOOD	AMOUNT	CALS	FAT (g.)
9" dia.	1/3 pie	550	31.3
Turnip, cooked:			
cubed	1 cup	36	.3
mashed	1 cup	53	.5
Turnip greens:			
canned	1 cup	42	.7
fresh, cooked	1 cup	29	.3
frozen, chopped,			
cooked	1 cup	38	.5

V

FOOD	AMOUNT	CALS	FAT (g.)
Veal, lean, trimmed, cooked:			
chuck and stew cuts	3 oz.	200	10.9
chuck and stew cuts,			
diced	1 cup	329	17.9
loin cuts	3 oz.	199	11.4
plate, breast	4 oz.	344	24.1
rib roast	3 oz.	229	14.4
rib roast, ground	1 cup	296	18.6
round with rump	3 oz.	184	9.4
Vegetable juice cocktail,			
canned	1 cup	41	.2
Vegetables, mixed, frozen,			
cooked	1 cup	116	.5
Venison, lean, uncooked	3 oz.	107	3.4
Vienna sausage (see Sausages)			
Vinegar:			
cider	1 tbsp.	2	0
distilled	1 tbsp.	2	0
Vodka (see Beverages)			

FOOD	AMOUNT	CALS	FAT (g.)

W

FOOD	AMOUNT	CALS	FAT (g.)
Waffles:			
from mix, round, 7" dia.	1	206	8.0
from mix, square, 4½"x4½"	1	138	5.3
frozen, 4⅝"x3¾"	1	86	2.1
homemade, round, 7" dia.	1	209	7.4
homemade, square, 4½"x4½"	1	140	4.9
Walnuts:			
black, shelled, chopped	1 tbsp.	50	4.7
Persian or English, in shell	10	322	31.7
Persian or English, shelled, halves	1 cup	651	64.0
Persian or English, shelled, chopped	1 tbsp.	52	5.1
Waterchestnuts, Chinese (matai)	1 oz.	17	t
Watercress, fresh:			
chopped	1 cup	24	.4
whole	1 cup	7	.1
Watermelon, fresh:			
diced	1 cup	42	.3
wedge	4" arc	111	.9
Welsh rarebit	1 cup	415	31.6
Wheat bran (see Flour)			
Wheat cereal (see Cereal)			
Wheat flour (see Flour)			
Wheat germ (see Cereal)			
Wheat parboiled (see Bulgur)			
Whey, fluid	1 cup	59	.2
Whiskey (see Beverages)			

FOOD	AMOUNT	CALS	FAT (g.)
Whitefish, lake, smoked	4 oz.	176	8.3
White sauce:			
thin	1 cup	303	21.8
medium	1 cup	405	31.3
thick	1 cup	495	39.0
Wine (see Beverages)			

Y

Yam, candied (see Potato, sweet)			
Yeast:			
bakers, compressed,			
.6 oz. cake	1	15	.1
bakers, dry, ¼ oz. pkg.	1	20	.1
brewer's, debittered	1 tbsp.	23	.1
torula	1 oz.	79	.3
Yogurt:			
from low-fat milk			
plain	8 oz.	144	3.5
from whole milk	8 oz.	139	7.8
Youngberries (see Blackberries)			

Z

Zucchini (see Squash, summer)
Zwieback (see Crackers)

THE PLANNING COUNTER

BREAKFAST FOOD SELECTIONS

Choose from the following *low calorie* foods to create your own delicious and nutritious breakfast menus. Note that all items contain no more than: *150 calories.* PER SERVING. Choose foods from the PROTEIN FOOD SELECTIONS section to further enhance your menus.

FOOD	AMOUNT	CALS	FAT (g.)
Applesauce:			
canned, unsweetened	1 cup	100	.5
Apricots:			
canned, unsweetened	1 cup	93	.2
fresh, halves	1 cup	79	.3
Banana:			
fresh, 7¾" long	1	81	.2
Blackberries:			
fresh	1 cup	84	1.3
frozen, unsweetened	1 cup	137	.4
Blueberries:			
fresh	1 cup	90	.7
frozen, unsweetened	1 cup	91	.8
Bread:			
cracked wheat	1 sl.	66	.6
French (2½" x 2" x ½")	1 sl.	44	.5
raisin	1 sl.	66	.7
rye	1 sl.	61	.3
whole wheat	1 sl.	67	.7
Cantaloupe:			
fresh, 5" dia.	1/2	82	.3
diced	1 cup	48	.2
Casaba melon:			
fresh, 7¾" long	1/10	38	1
Cereal:			
puffed rice	1 cup	60	.1

FOOD	AMOUNT	CALS	FAT (g.)
puffed wheat	1 cup	54	.2
shredded wheat	1 biscuit	89	.5
wheat germ	1 tbsp.	23	.7
Cocoa powder,			
medium fat	1 tbsp.	14	1.0
Cranberries, fresh, whole	1 cup	44	.7
Cream substitute,			
non-dairy	1 tbsp.	20	1.5
Fruit salad:			
canned, unsweetened	1 cup	86	.2
Grapefruit:			
canned, unsweetened	1 cup	73	.2
fresh, 3-9/16" dia.	1/2	40	.1
fresh, sections	1 cup	82	.2
Guava, fresh	1 med.	48	t
Margarine, regular	1 pat	36	4.1
Milk, skim	1 cup	86	.4
Nectarines, fresh, 2½" dia.	1	88	t
Oranges, fresh:			
Navel, 2⅞" dia.	1	71	.1
sections	1 cup	88	.4
Papaya, fresh, cubed	1 cup	55	.1
Peanut butter,			
commercial	1 tbsp.	94	8.1
Pineapple, canned,			
unsweetened, cuts*	1 cup	96	.2
Prunes, dried, large	1	22	t
Raisins, seedless, whole	1 tbsp.	26	t
Raspberries, fresh:			
black	1 cup	98	1.9
red	1 cup	70	.6

*chunk, tidbit, crushed
*Varies, depending on type; can equal zero

FOOD	AMOUNT	CALS	FAT (g.)
Strawberries, fresh, whole	1 cup	55	.7
Tangelo, fresh, 2¾" dia.	1	47	.1
Tangerine, fresh:			
2½" dia.	1	46	.2
sections	1 cup	90	.4

LUNCH and DINNER FOOD SELECTIONS

Choose from the following *low calorie* foods to create
your own delicious and nutritious lunch and dinner menus.
Note that all items contain no more than: *150 calories* PER
SERVING. Choose foods from the PROTEIN FOOD
SELECTIONS section to further enhance your menus.

FOOD	AMOUNT	CALS	FAT (g.)
Artichokes:			
French or Globe,			
cooked	1 bud	16	.2
Jerusalem, pared,			
cooked	4 oz.	75	.2
Asparagus:			
fresh, spears, cooked	1 cup	36	.4
Bamboo shoots, fresh	1 cup	41	.5
Beans:			
green or snap,			
fresh, cooked	1 cup	31	.3
French style,			

FOOD	AMOUNT	CALS	FAT (g.)
frozen, cooked	1 cup	34	.1
sprouts, mung	1 cup	37	.2
yellow or wax,			
frozen, cooked	1 cup	36	.1
Beets, fresh, diced or			
sliced	1 cup	54	.2
Beet greens, cooked	1 cup	26	.3
Boston brown bread:			
canned, ½" thick	1 sl.	95	.6
Bread:			
cracked wheat	1 sl.	66	.6
French (2½" x 2" x ½")	1 sl.	44	.5
raisin	1 sl.	66	.7
rye	1 sl.	61	.3
whole wheat	1 sl.	67	.7
Breadsticks, 4½" long	1	38	.3
Broccoli:			
fresh, stalks	1 med.	47	.5
frozen, chopped,			
cooked	1 cup	48	.6
Brussels sprouts:			
frozen, cooked	1 cup	51	.3
Cabbage:			
white, wedges, cooked	1 cup	31	.3
Cake, from mix:			
angel food, cubed	1 cu. in.	6	t
cupcake, uniced, 2½" dia.	1	88	3.0
Carrots:			
fresh, 7" long	1	30	.1
fresh, sliced, cooked	1 cup	48	.3
Cauliflower:			
fresh, whole buds	1 cup	27	.2
frozen, cooked	1 cup	32	.4
Celery, fresh, 8" long	1 stalk	7	

FOOD	AMOUNT	CALS	FAT (g.)
Chard, Swiss, fresh, cooked	1 cup	26	.3
Cheese straws, 5" long	1	27	1.8
Cherries, sour, fresh:			
whole (pitted)	1 cup	90	.5
Collards:			
fresh, cooked	1 cup	63	1.3
frozen, chopped, cooked	1 cup	51	.7
Cookies:			
butter thins, 2" dia.	1	23	.9
graham crackers, plain	2" sq.	28	.7
Corn, fresh:			
on the cob, cooked	5" ear	70	.8
Crackers:			
butter, round, 1⅞" dia.	1	15	.6
rye wafers, 3½" x 1⅞"	1	22	t
soda, 1⅞" sq.	1	12	.4
soda, biscuit, 2⅜" x 2⅛"	1	22	.7
wheat thins	4	55	3.1
zwieback, 3½" x 1½"	1	30	.6
Cress, garden, cooked	1 cup	31	.8
Cucumber, peeled, sliced	1 cup	20	.1
Dandilion greens, cooked	1 cup	35	.6
Endive, fresh, chopped	1 cup	10	.1
Fruit cocktail:			
canned, unsweetened	1 cup	91	.2
Fruit salad:			
canned, unsweetened	1 cup	86	.2
Kale:			
fresh, cooked	1 cup	43	.8
frozen, cooked	1 cup	40	.7

FOOD	AMOUNT	CALS	FAT (g.)
Kohlrabi, fresh:			
diced, cooked	1 cup	40	.2
Lettuce, raw:			
iceberg, wedge	1/4 head	18	.1
romaine, chopped	1 cup	10	.2
Mushrooms, fresh:			
chopped or sliced	1 cup	20	.2
Mustard greens:			
fresh, cooked	1 cup	32	.6
frozen, chopped, cooked	1 cup	30	.6
Okra:			
fresh, sliced, cooked	1 cup	46	.5
frozen, sliced, cooked	1 cup	70	.2
Onions:			
green, tops only, chopped (scallions)	1 tbsp.	2	t
mature, whole or sliced, cooked	1 cup	61	.2
Parsley, fresh, whole sprigs	10	4	.1
Parsnips:			
cooked, whole, 6" long	1	23	.2
Peaches:			
canned, unsweetened	1 cup	76	.2
fresh, 2½" dia.	1	38	.1
Peanut butter, commercial	1 tbsp.	94	8.1
Pears:			
canned, unsweetened	1 cup	78	.5
fresh, Bartlett, 2½" dia.	1	100	.7
fresh, Bosc, 2½" dia.	1	86	.6
Peppers, sweet:			
green, 3" dia	1 ring	2	t
green, sliced	1 cup	18	.2

FOOD	AMOUNT	CALS	FAT (g.)
red, 3" dia.	1 ring	3	t
Pickles, sweet:			
chopped	1 tbsp.	15	t
gherkin, midget	1	9	t
mustard			
(Chow-chow)	1 tbsp.	18	.1
Pineapple:			
canned, unsweetened,			
cuts*	1 cup	96	.2
fresh, sliced, 3½" dia.	1	44	.2
Plums, fresh:			
Damson, 1" dia.	10	66	t
Japanese, diced	1 cup	79	.3
prune-type, 1½" dia.	1	21	.1
Raisins, seedless, whole	1 tbsp.	26	t
Rhubarb, fresh, diced	1 cup	20	.1
Rutabagas:			
fresh, cooked, mashed	1 cup	84	.2
Salad dressings, commercial:			
French, low-calorie	1 tbsp.	15	.7
Italian, low-calorie	1 tbsp.	8	.7
Russian, low-calorie	1 tbsp.	23	.7
Salad dressing			
(mayonnaise-type)	1 tbsp.	65	6.3
Salad dressing,			
low-calorie	1 tbsp.	22	2.0
Thousand Island,			
low-calorie	1 tbsp.	27	2.1
Soybean curd (tofu),			
2½" x 2¾"	1 piece	86	5.0
sprouts	1 cup	48	1.5

*chunks, crushed, tidbits

FOOD	AMOUNT	CALS	FAT (g.)
Spinach:			
fresh, chopped .... 1 cup		14	.2
frozen, leaf, cooked .... 1 cup		46	.6
Squash, summer:			
fresh, cooked, sliced .... 1 cup		29	.2
Squash, winter, fresh:			
acorn, baked, 4" dia. 1/2		86	.2
butternut, boiled,			
mashed .... 1 cup		100	.2
hubbard, boiled, diced .... 1 cup		71	.7
Tomatoes:			
fresh, 2-3/5" dia. 1		27	.2
fresh, cooked .... 1 cup		63	.5
Turnip, cooked, mashed .... 1 cup		53	.5
Turnip greens:			
frozen, chopped,			
cooked .... 1 cup		38	.5
Waterchestnuts, Chinese .... 1 oz.		17	t
Watercress, fresh,			
chopped .... 1 cup		24	.4
Watermelon, fresh, diced .... 1 cup		42	.3

SNACK SELECTIONS

Choose from the following *low calorie* foods to create your own delicious and nutritious snacks. Note that all items contain no more than: *150 calories* PER SERVING. Choose foods from the PROTEIN FOOD SELECTIONS section to further enhance your snacks.

FOOD	AMOUNT	CALS	FAT (g.)
Apples, fresh, whole, 3" dia. 1		96	1.0
Applesauce:			
canned, unsweetened .... 1 cup		100	.5

FOOD	AMOUNT	CALS	FAT (g.)
Apricots, fresh, whole	3	55	.2
Banana, fresh, 7¾" long	1	81	.2
Blackberries, fresh	1 cup	84	1.3
Blueberries, fresh	1 cup	90	.7
Breadsticks, 4½" long	1	38	.3
Cake, from mix:			
angel food, cubed	1 cu. in.		t
Celery, fresh, 8" long	1 stalk	7	t
Cherries, sour, fresh,			
whole (pitted)	1 cup	90	.5
Crackers:			
butter, round, 1⅞" dia.	1	15	.6
rye wafers, 3½" x 1⅞"	1	22	t
soda, 1⅞" sq.	1	12	.4
soda, biscuit, 2⅜" x 2⅛"	1	22	.7
wheat thins	4	55	3.1
zwieback, 3½" x 1½"	1	30	.6
Fig:			
dried	1	55	.2
fresh, 2¼" dia.	1	40	.2
Gooseberries, fresh	1 cup	59	.3
Granadilla (Passion fruit),			
fresh	1	16	.1
Grapefruit, fresh,			
3-9/16" dia.	1/2	40	.1
Grapes, fresh,			
American-type	1 cup	70	1.0
Guava, fresh	1 med.	48	t
Kumquat, fresh	1 sm.	15	t
Loganberries, fresh	1 cup	89	.9
Lychees, fresh	10	58	.3
Margarine, regular	1 pat	36	4.1
Nectarines, fresh, 2½" dia.	1	88	t
Oranges, fresh, Navel, 2⅞" dia.	1	71	.1

118

FOOD	AMOUNT	CALS	FAT (g.)
Papaya, fresh, cubed	1 cup	55	.1
Peaches, fresh:			
2½" dia.	1	38	.1
diced	1 cup	70	.2
Peanut butter,			
commercial	1 tbsp.	94	8.1
Peanuts, roasted, shell,			
jumbo	10	105	8.8
Pears, fresh:			
Bartlett, 2½" dia.	1	100	.7
Bosc, 2½" dia.	1	86	.6
Peppers, sweet:			
green, 3" dia.	1 ring	2	t
red, 3" dia.	1 ring	3	t
Pickles, sweet:			
chopped	1 tbsp.	15	t
gherkin midget	1	9	t
mustard			
(Chow-chow)	1 tbsp.	18	.1
Pineapple:			
canned, unsweetened			
cuts**	1 cup	96	.2
fresh, sliced, 3½" dia.	1	44	.2
Plums, fresh:			
Damson, 1" dia.	10	66	t
Japanese, 2⅛" dia.	1	32	.1
prune-type, 1½" dia.	1	21	.1
Pomegranate, fresh, 3⅜" dia.	1	97	.5
Popcorn, plain	1 cup	23	.3
Prunes, dried, large	1	22	t
Radishes, fresh, large	10	14	.1
Raisins, seedless, whole	1 tbsp.	26	t

**chunks, crushed, tidbits

FOOD	AMOUNT	CALS	FA [g]
Raspberries, fresh:			
black	1 cup	98	1.9
red	1 cup	70	.6
Rusk, 3⅜" dia.	1	38	.8
Strawberries, fresh, whole	1 cup	55	.7
Tangelo, fresh, 2¾" dia.	1	47	.1
Tangerine, fresh, 2½" dia.	1	46	.2

BEVERAGE SELECTIONS

Choose from the following *low-calorie* beverages at meals or snacks. Note that all items contain no more than: 120 calories PER SERVING.

Apple juice, canned or bottled	1 cup	117	t
Beverages, alcoholic:			
beer, "light"	12 oz.	96	t
wine, table (12% alcohol)	3½ oz.	87	0
Beverages, carbonated:			
club soda, unsweetened	12 oz.	0	0
tonic water	12 oz.	113	0
Blackberry juice, canned, unsweetened	1 cup	91	1.5
Cocoa:			
beverage powder	1 oz.	98	.8
medium-fat powder	1 tbsp.	14	1.0
Coffee, prepared, plain	1 cup	2	
Grapefruit juice:			
canned, unsweetened	1 cup	101	.2
fresh	1 cup	96	.2

FOOD	AMOUNT	CALS	FAT (g.)
Grapefruit-orange juice, canned			
unsweetened	1 cup	106	.5
Lemonade, frozen,			
sweetened	1 cup	107	t
Limeade, frozen,			
sweetened	1 cup	102	t
Milk:			
low-fat, 2%	1 cup	121	4.7
skim	1 cup	86	.4
Orange juice:			
fresh	1 cup	112	.5
frozen, unsweetened	1 cup	114	.7
Tangelo juice, fresh	1 cup	101	.2
Tangerine juice:			
canned, unsweetened	1 cup	106	.5
fresh	1 cup	106	.5

PROTEIN FOOD SELECTIONS

Choose from the following *low calorie* protein foods to enhance your meals and snacks. Note that all items contain no more than: *200 calories* PER SERVING. In moderate amounts, these nutritious foods provide ample protein without contributing excessive amounts of *calories*.

BREAKFAST SELECTIONS:

FOOD	AMOUNT	CALS	FAT (g.)
Cottage cheese,			
uncreamed	1 cup	123	.6
Milk:			
low fat, 2%	1 cup	121	4.7
skim	1 cup	86	.4
Sardines, Atlantic, canned,			
3" long	1	24	1.3

FOOD	AMOUNT	CALS	FAT (g.)
Sausage, pork, fresh,			
cooked	1 link	62	5.7
Yogurt, from lowfat milk,			
plain	8 oz.	144	3.5

LUNCH and DINNER SELECTIONS:

FOOD	AMOUNT	CALS	FAT (g.)
Beef, lean, trimmed, cooked:			
chuck, roast or steak	3 oz.	164	6.0
flank steak			
(London broil)	3 oz.	167	6.2
ground, 10% fat	3 oz.	186	9.6
round steak	3 oz.	161	5.2
rump roast	3 oz.	177	7.9
sirloin, double-bone	3 oz.	184	8.1
sirloin wedge- and			
round-bone	3 oz.	176	6.5
Bluefish, fresh, baked with			
margarine	4 oz.	185	5.9
Cheese:			
Brie	1 oz.	95	7.9
Brick	1 oz.	105	8.4
Cheddar, domestic	1 oz.	114	9.4
Colby	1 oz.	112	9.1
Cottage, uncreamed	1 cup	123	.6
Mozzarella, part-skim	1 oz.	72	4.5
Muenster	1 oz.	104	8.5
Neufchatel	1 oz.	74	6.6
Parmesan, grated	1 tbsp.	23	1.5
Swiss, domestic	1 oz.	107	7.8
Chicken:			
broiler	3 oz.	116	3.2
roaster	3 oz.	156	5.5
Cod, fresh, broiled with			

FOOD	AMOUNT	CALS	FAT (g.)
margarine	4 oz.	192	6.0
Goose, domesticated, cooked	3 oz.	198	8.3
Haddock, fresh, oven-fried	4 oz.	188	7.2
Halibut, fresh, broiled with margarine	4 oz.	192	8.0
Ham:			
boiled	1 oz.	66	4.8
deviled, canned	1 tbsp.	46	4.2
fresh	3 oz.	184	8.5
fresh shoulder pork (Picnic)	3 oz.	180	8.3
Rockfish, fresh, cooked	4 oz.	24	2.0
Sardines, Atlantic, canned, 3" long	1	204	1.3
Smelt, fresh	7 med.	100	—
Sole, fresh, cooked	4 oz.	90	—
Swordfish, fresh, broiled with margarine	4 oz.	184	6.4
Tongue, beef, cooked	2 oz.	138	9.5
Tuna:			
canned in water	4 oz.	144	.9
fresh, cooked	3 oz.	105	—
Turkey, cooked, light meat	3 oz.	150	3.3

SNACK SELECTIONS:

FOOD	AMOUNT	CALS	FAT (g.)
Almonds, dried, shelled, chopped	1 tbsp.	48	4.3
Brazil nuts, shelled, large	6	185	19.0
Cheese (see Lunch and Dinner Selections above)			
Cheese straws, 5" long	1	27	1.8
Chestnuts, in shell	10	141	1.1
Filberts	10	87	8.6
Ham, boiled	1 oz.	66	4.8
Ice milk, plain, 5% fat	1 cup	184	5.6
Pecans, shelled, chopped	1 tbsp.	52	5.3
Sardines, Atlantic, canned, 3" long	1	24	1.3
Walnuts, shelled, chopped	1 tbsp.	52	5.1
Yogurt, from lowfat milk, plain	8 oz.	144	3.5

APPENDIX: COMMON MEASUREMENTS CONVERSION TABLE

Use the table below to assist you in converting given quantities of foods into the desired equivalents.

5 milliliters	= 1 teaspoon
3 teaspoons	= 1 tablespoon
16 tablespoons	= 1 cup = 8 fluid ounces
2 cups	= 1 pint = 16 fluid ounces
2 pints	= 1 quart = 32 fluid ounces
4 quarts	= 1 gallon = 128 fluid ounces
28.35 grams	= 1 ounce = 2 fluid tablespoons
16 ounces	= 1 pound = 453.6 grams
8 quarts	= 1 peck
4 pecks	= 1 bushel

APPENDIX: METRIC CONVERSION TABLE

The U.S. Department of Agriculture uses the following rounded figures for converting quantities of foods, energy values, and temperatures into metric system equivalents:

U.S. SYSTEM	Metric System Equivalent
	Length:
1 inch	2.54 centimeters,
	25.4 millimeters
	Volume:
1 cubic inch	16.39 cubic centimeters
1 teaspoon	5 milliliters
1 tablespoon	15 milliliters
1 fluid ounce	30 milliliters
1 cup	240 milliliters
1 pint	475 milliliters
1 quart	950 milliliters
1 gallon	3.8 liters
	Energy:
1 kilocalorie	4.184 kiloJoules
	Temperature:
1° Fahrenheit (F)	5/9° Celsius (C)

APPENDIX:

DESIRED WEIGHTS (without clothing)

Women Height (Without Shoes)	Small Frame	Medium Frame	Large Frame
5 ft. 0 in.	92- 98	96-107	104-109
5 ft. 1 in.	94-101	98-110	106-112
5 ft. 2 in.	96-104	101-112	109-118
5 ft. 3 in.	99-107	104-116	112-121
5 ft. 4 in.	102-110	107-119	115-125
5 ft. 5 in.	105-113	110-122	118-130
5 ft. 6 in.	108-116	113-126	121-135
5 ft. 7 in.	111-119	116-130	125-140
5 ft. 8 in.	114-123	120-135	129-145
5 ft. 9 in.	118-127	124-139	133-150
5 ft. 10 in.	122-131	128-143	137-155
5 ft. 11 in.	126-135	132-147	141-160
6 ft. 0 in.	130-140	136-151	145-165
Men			
5 ft. 4 in.	115-123	121-133	129-132
5 ft. 5 in.	118-126	124-136	132-137
5 ft. 6 in.	121-129	127-139	135-142
5 ft. 7 in.	124-133	130-143	138-148
5 ft. 8 in.	128-137	134-147	142-152
5 ft. 9 in.	132-141	138-152	147-155
5 ft. 10 in.	136-145	142-156	151-160
5 ft. 11 in.	140-150	146-160	155-165
6 ft. 0 in.	144-154	150-165	159-170
6 ft. 1 in.	148-158	154-170	164-175
6 ft. 2 in.	152-162	158-175	168-180
6 ft. 3 in.	156-167	162-180	173-185
6 ft. 4 in.	160-171	167-185	178-190

Note: Prepared by the Metropolitan Life Insurance Company. Derived primarily from data of the Build and Blood Pressure Study, 1959, Society of Actuaries.

Diet Diary

Diet Diary